THE STRETCHING BIBLE

THE STRETCHING BIBLE

THE ULTIMATE GUIDE TO IMPROVING FITNESS & FLEXIBILITY

LEXIE WILLIAMSON

BLOOMSBURY

LONDON · OXFORD · NEW YORK · NEW DELHI · SYDNEY

Bloomsbury Sport
An imprint of Bloomsbury Publishing Plc

50 Bedford Square	1385 Broadway
London	New York
WC1B 3DP	NY 10018
UK	USA

www.bloomsbury.com

BLOOMSBURY and the Diana logo are trademarks
of Bloomsbury Publishing Plc

First published in 2017
© Lexie Williamson, 2017
Photos by Grant Pritchard Photography
Photos on page 148–149 © Getty Images

A catalogue record for this book is available from
the British Library.

ISBN: Paperback: 9781472929877
         ePub: 9781472929884
         ePDF: 9781472929891

2 4 6 8 10 9 7 5 3 1

Typeset in Aptifer Sans and Slab by seagulls.net
Printed and bound in China by C&C Offset Printing Co.

Bloomsbury Publishing Plc makes every effort to
ensure that the papers used in the manufacture
of our books are natural, recyclable products
made from wood grown in well-managed forests.
Our manufacturing processes conform to the
environmental regulations of the country of origin.

To find out more about our authors and books visit
www.bloomsbury.com. Here you will find extracts,
author interviews, details of forthcoming events and
the option to sign up for our newsletters.

CONTENTS

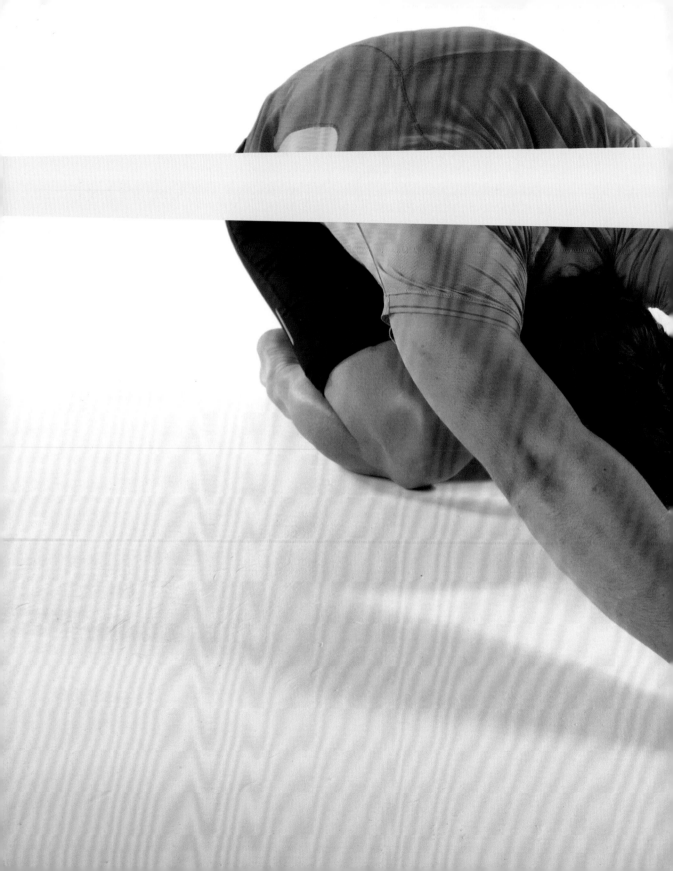

Introduction

There are 101 Reasons to Stretch

To sit straighter, stand taller, move more freely, sidestep injury, release stress, feel younger, improve your golf swing and sleep better.

The Stretching Bible is a one-stop resource that packages stretches and ready-made sequences in a way that is easy and accessible – whatever your reasons for wanting to be more supple or mobile. It offers sequences for different ages, (children, teenagers and seniors), occupations (commuters, desk workers and manual workers), time constraints (five minute routines), and level (gentle, intermediate and advanced).

Stretching techniques are also divided into anatomical sections, such as for your back and sides or your upper legs, in order to hone in on exercises for an aching lower back, tight hamstrings or stiff shoulders. And the final section features highly targeted warm-up and cool down stretching routines for 20 sports from American football through to weight training.

In the last few years of bringing sport-specific yoga to athletes as a Yoga Sports Coach™, I've witnessed a tenfold increase in interest within the sports community in what we call 'flexibility training'. The emphasis for athletes is not on replicating pretzel positions (although advanced stretches are here for those wishing to go deeper), but on simple, functional techniques to improve performance and reduce post-exercise muscle soreness.

Of course, the global rise in popularity of yoga and Pilates demonstrates that many people also want to stretch simply because it feels good. Some have sedentary desk jobs and need to move and release muscular tension. Others are seeking a little mental and physical 'space' in a stressful world. Regardless of age, occupation, situation and perceived flexibility levels there are a range of stretches to suit everyone, so flick through, experiment and enjoy.

Why Stretch?
To counter the desk job

Many of us now spend eight, nine or ten hours a day at our desks. Add in time spent commuting and these long periods of sitting can negatively impact the body. Possibly the biggest side effect of prolonged sitting is lower back pain and discomfort. Simple stretches will maintain comfort levels throughout the day and lessen the effect of sedentary work. Many are so simple and subtle that co-workers won't even notice that you are stretching. *See The Desk Worker sequence (page 114).*

To maintain mobility in old age

Our range of motion can (but doesn't have to) lessen gradually over the years, and these physiological changes, combined with a reduction in activity, result in stiffer joints, but a good level of flexibility can be maintained with a regular stretching routine. Many of my best yoga students are older ladies who outshine me on the mat with their strong, supple bodies: the product of a lifetime of stretching. Having said that, it's never too late to start stretching. The emphasis is not on touching toes or forcing the body into gymnastic shapes but on gentle, limbering movements to improve blood flow, increase energy and help facilitate everyday movements.

See Stretching for Seniors sequence, page 128.

To avoid injury

Ten-minute stretches post-run or bike ride, or after non-athletic endeavours such as clearing snow or mowing the lawn, will greatly reduce the chance of injury. This is stretching as pre-habilitation or 'pre-hab' rather than 'rehab' (for which a physiotherapist should be your first port of call). Sportspeople know they *ought* to stretch, but are sometimes unsure what stretches to try for their sport or become stuck in a rut repeating a routine that is not sport-specific. Aside from helping sportspeople avoid injury, stretching can vastly reduce the chances of suffering with DOMS (Delayed Onset Muscle Soreness) or that inability to bend your knees to descend the stairs 24 to 48 hours after a squat-heavy gym session.

See Stretches by Sport section (page 164).

To improve posture

Modern life demands that we sit a lot while driving, commuting, working at a desk or relaxing on the sofa, and the temptation to slouch is ever-present. Gravity and time also play a part in poor posture. But a few simple stretches, combined with a little back strengthening, can remedy this and result in a healthier, more upright stance that feels good and conveys

confidence. Many are simple movements, such as drawing back the shoulders and squeezing the shoulder blades closer, but will gradually instill an everyday awareness of how we are sitting or standing. Stretching can make a huge difference to posture, especially when combined with back-strengthening exercises such as the Cobra on page 54.

See the Better Posture sequence (page 122).

To relieve stress

Stress is essentially a mental phenomenon and usually the result of a perceived inability to cope with life's demands, but the effects are partly physical: gritted teeth, a churning stomach and muscles that feel 'locked' particularly around the shoulders. Stretching unlocks this muscular tightness. Gentle movements, such as head rolls or relaxing stretches, calm the mind. This soothing effect is doubled when stretching is combined with deep breathing. Many people in the West now flock to yoga as it releases stress through a system of physical stretching and breathing. Novice yoga students sometimes proceed to mental control through meditation techniques, but the majority just enjoy the simple pleasure of lying on a mat, reaching their arms overhead and other physical stretches.

See The Stress Reducer (page 132).

To combat insomnia

It is thought that one in three of us suffer with insomnia and most of us experience bouts of wakefulness at stressful times of our lives. A regular pre-bedtime stretching sequence can be part of a winding down process and help reduce the stress, which may be at the root of the insomnia. These stretches can be used both to encourage the onset of sleep and instigate a return to sleep if insomnia strikes in the early hours of the morning. They are termed 'passive stretches', meaning that they require no balance or strength to perform, and focus on relaxation.

See The Pre-Bed Relaxer sequence (page 134).

Improve athletic performance

Picture a golfer coiling the upper body back in preparation to swing through, a soccer player diving for the ball or a weight lifter sinking into a deep squat and it is clear that flexibility can improve power. It is true to say that you cannot boost power with stretching alone, but a combination of flexibility and strength training can reap huge benefits for amateur and professional sportspeople. Improved flexibility can also help athletes achieve the physical positions they desire, whether they are triathletes tucking low on the bike to avoid drag or tennis players lunging sideways to reach a shot.

See the Stretching for Sport section and find your sport (pages 164).

Types of Stretching

There is a confusing array of stretching types, but, for ease and clarity, this book largely features two types: 'static' and 'dynamic' with a few 'assisted' stretches, or those requiring a partner. Used together, static and dynamic techniques can improve the two components of flexibility: muscle length and joint range of motion.

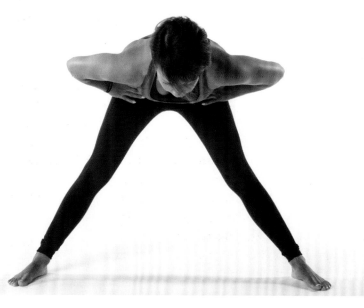

Static

When people talk of stretching they are generally referring to static stretching or holding a stretch without movement. While it may not have the dramatic returns promised by other forms of stretching, it is thought to be the safest form. The muscles are relaxed and then stretched through holding twisting, forward bending or back bending positions. The muscle is slowly lengthened to the point of tension or to the 'edge' of the stretch. Bouncing or jerking movements, such as sitting with the soles of your feet together and flapping your knees up and down, can actually make the muscle contract, achieving the exact opposite of what is desired. The same contracting response can occur when we push hard into a stretch. Shaking and grimacing are often signals of too much, too soon. If this occurs when you stretch, back off, breathe slowly and deeply and start again.

Dynamic

The term 'dynamic' is a loose one, but in this book it refers to controlled and rhythmic movements mostly used during the warm-up sections. These movements are gentle, slow and within the person's normal joint range of motion. They are comfortable and simple, for example, swinging a leg back and forth or rolling the shoulders. The main aim is to raise the heart rate slightly and encourage blood flow to the part of the body that you either intend to stretch deeper or involve in athletic endeavours.

HOW LONG SHOULD I HOLD A STRETCH?

According to studies, 30 seconds is the ideal amount of time to hold a stretch. Beyond this, little more is gained in terms of flexibility. Of course, this depends who you talk to. Sports scientists would probably say 20-30 seconds while some schools of yoga hold postures for three minutes. I think it depends on what you've done prior to stretching and which muscle group you are targeting. For example, a minute would seem like a long time to stretch the delicate neck muscles if they are a little stiff, but you can hold a stretch for the larger, thicker muscles of the hips after a long bike ride and still deepen the stretch after two minutes. If you are stretching to aid relaxation, you may also want to hold for longer; this is reflected in the pre-bed and stress-releasing sequences later in the book.

Sportspeople can also select dynamic movements that mimic their sport, thereby ingraining movement patterns in their minds before actually picking up a racquet or running on the track. These movements can be made faster and more dynamic by adding skipping or walking, but only if the athlete has no injuries and takes care.

Do you need to warm up or do dynamic stretches before holding static stretches? It will only help, especially if you feel very stiff, are largely sedentary or are elderly. Warm muscles respond better to stretching.

Assisted or partner

The *Stretches by Sport* section contains some techniques done with the aid of a partner, either performing the stretch together or taking turns to lengthen one another's muscles. Work with a partner you trust and communicate continually during the stretching process. If you are the one assisting, regularly ask your partner how they feel and look for signs of discomfort (such as grimacing) which may mean you are pushing too quickly or too far. Partner stretching is also a great means of forging bonds between sports team members.

What Determines Flexibility?

The degree of flexibility you possess is determined by a number of factors some of which (like genetics) are out of your control. Therefore, the type of stretch you choose depends on your body. One person's 'advanced' stretch might be another's 'gentle'. Never try to mimic a photograph of an advanced stretch if it doesn't suit you physically or causes discomfort or pain. It cannot be stressed enough: all that matters is that you feel the correct muscles lengthening.

Flexibility is determined by a number of factors, including:

- **Sex** Women have greater range of motion than men at the hips, knees and ankles,

> ## WHAT IS FLEXIBILITY?
>
> The term flexibility refers to achieving full range of motion around a joint, for example, being able to rotate your ball-and-socket shoulder joint freely across 365 degrees when 'rolling' your shoulder. Full range of motion is ideal as it allows joints to adapt to stress imposed on the body and decreases the potential for injury. A good motto for range of motion is 'move it, or lose it.' To achieve it, we need to target both joint range of motion (the motion available at the joint) and muscle length (the ability of a muscle crossing the joint to lengthen). The techniques in this book target both joint range of motion with dynamic head rolling or leg swinging-type techniques and muscle length through static or long-held stretching.

according to research. Studies comparing upper body mobility between the sexes, such as shoulder range of motion, are less conclusive, showing females have superior range of motion in some planes while men excel in others.

- **Age** Muscles can become stiffer as we age as do the supporting ligaments and tendons, but decreased activity may also be a major reason that we lose mobility. There is also less lubricating joint fluid. However, stretching and other activity gradually improves lubrication until movement becomes easier. 'An analogy is [that of] applying a drop of oil to a stubborn

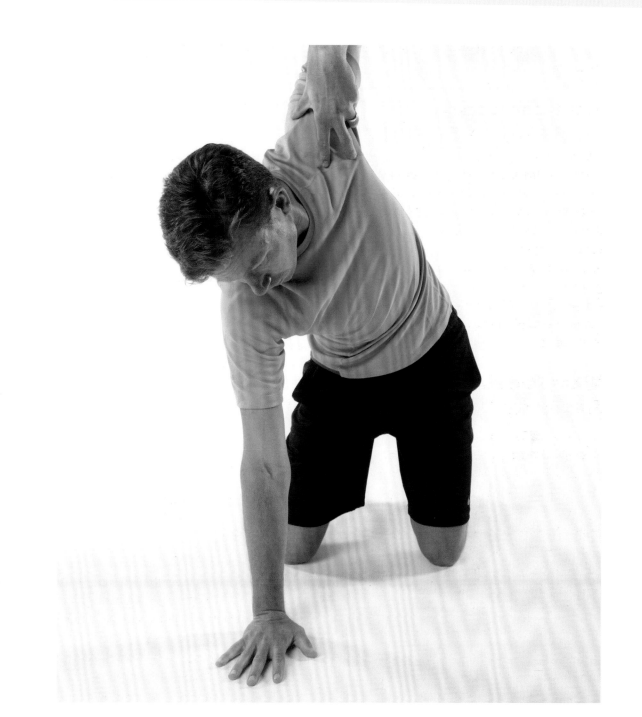

SEVEN RULES FOR SAFE STRETCHING

Just like with any other activity, it is possible to damage muscles by stretching, usually by pushing too hard or too fast. Follow these seven simple rules to ensure your stretching regime works for, not against, you.

1 Don't stretch cold muscles Brisk walking or limbering movements, such as making circular movements with the arms, will raise the body temperature and make the muscles more pliable and responsive to stretching.

2 Don't push too far, too soon Muscles will contract in response to quick, aggressive stretching, creating exactly the opposite effect to lengthening. Begin at the 'edge' of the stretch by experiencing a light tension then gradually deepen over time. This way you override the body's natural 'contract to protect' mechanism.

3 Stretching shouldn't hurt Grimacing and shaking should not be visible when stretching. Again, this will only trigger the body's safety mechanisms and cause the muscles to tighten further.

4 Get expert advice regarding injuries Stretching is a fantastic way of preventing common overuse injuries but may not be part of a rehabilitation plan. Check with your physiotherapist or medical practitioner before embarking on stretches that target your injured area.

5 Stay for 20-60 seconds For some, having the patience to hold a static stretch can be challenging, but standing on one leg, lifting the other and doing a cursory five-second tug will not lengthen the thighs, or quadriceps, after a run. Spend 20-60 seconds holding a stretch or follow a more dynamic sequence that keeps the muscles moving and holds your interest.

6 Don't forget to breathe Slow, deep breathing aids the stretching process by triggering the body's parasympathetic 'rest and restore' response – the opposite of the heightened 'fight or flight'. This relaxes muscles, which, in turn, aids stretching. If deep breathing is new to you, just breathe slower and through your nose.

7 Exit slowly Take your time to come out of the stretch particularly if you've held the position for over a minute as exiting quickly might injure the lower back. This is particularly relevant to standing or sitting forward-bending movements often used to stretch the hamstrings.

gate and then opening and closing it until it stops squeaking,' explains Dr Mark S. Lachs, Director of the Centre for Aging Research and Clinical Care at the Weill Medical College of Cornell University.

- **Genetics** The composition of elastin and collagen in the connective tissue is determined by birth. This explains why some people seem to be naturally supple. However, through regular and diligent stretching it is possible to improve the elastic quality of muscles and improve flexibility. In my experience, the people who become visibly more supple in the fastest time stretch at least three or four times a week.

- **Body Proportions** A man with broad shoulders may struggle to do some advanced shoulder stretches and this is simply a matter of body shape. The problem can usually be circumvented with the use of stretching aids, such as straps. Possessing shorter legs and a

WHEN SHOULD I STRETCH?

Whenever you remember: waiting for the kettle to boil, in the shower or while watching T.V. Some people like to stretch in the morning while others favour a post-work stretching routine to de-stress and relax. Stretch before and after exercise, but do gentle, limbering movements beforehand and save the longer-held or static stretches for after the workout. Little and often is ideal, but do what you can.

HOW FLEXIBLE AM I?

It's too easy to label yourself as 'supple' or 'stiff', but the truth is most people are a bit of both, depending on what area of the body they are stretching. You may struggle to touch your toes, but show superior hip flexibility by lying on your back – frog-like – with your legs bent and soles of your feet together. Therefore, flexibility must be seen as specific to a particular joint or muscle. There is a baffling array of tests which measure flexibility if you are serious about measuring progress. Otherwise, simply work within your limits and enjoy stretching for the many benefits it provides.

long torso also simply means that it's easier to do certain stretches such as reaching for your toes when sitting or standing. This doesn't mean that the owner of this type of body does not still need to stretch their hamstrings – they just make it look easy.

Stretching Aids and Equipment

A simple tool such as an old tie, dressing gown belt or purpose-made cotton yoga strap can open up a world of new stretches for those with limited flexibility, letting you move into the correct position. A classic example of this is the seated hamstring stretch where the legs are straightened out and the person stretching leans forwards to touch their toes. For more than half the population, this will simply result in stretching the lower back. By looping a strap around the soles of the feet and sitting more upright, the stretch shifts to the correct muscles: the hamstrings at the back of the thighs. You may also benefit from sitting on the edge of a cushion or a yoga foam block. This tilts the pelvis forwards, which, again, takes the pressure off the back. I liberally distribute straps and blocks during yoga sessions to account for levels of flexibility and recommend using both to anyone with limited range of motion. Here are a few useful aids.

Stretching aid 1: strap

Straps can be used in various ways such as looping around the feet in seated hamstring stretches or aiding shoulder stretches. You don't need to buy a purpose-made cotton yoga strap as an old tie or dressing gown belt makes a good substitute.

Here are three examples of strap usage:

1 **Lying Hamstring Strap Stretch** Looping a strap around the sole of the foot makes this

classic hamstring stretch accessible for everyone, however resistant the muscles. The intensity of the stretch can also be altered by walking your hands up the strap to draw the leg closer, or releasing an inch or two to let the leg move away.

2 **Overhead Strap Stretch** A strap provides an easy way to 'open' your chest and lengthen

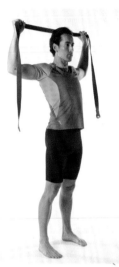

upper chest muscles including pectoralis major and minor – a great feeling particularly if you have been slouched over a computer, driving or riding a bike.

3 **Lying Quad Stretch** If you find yourself reaching in vain for the foot in this face down front-of-thigh stretch, try hooking a strap around the ankle, holding on to both parts of the strap and gently drawing the heel in towards the buttocks. Or use a strap in the standing version of this stretch.

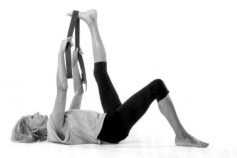

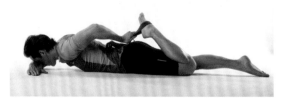

Stretching aid 2: foam block or cushion

The main purpose of a yoga foam block or household cushion is to make seated stretches more comfortable, especially for those with tight hamstrings, a stiff back or lower back problems. They can also make the cross-legged position more accessible.

Here are three examples of foam block or cushion usage:

1 **Seated Hamstring Stretch** If all you feel is lower back strain in a seated hamstring stretch, try perching on the edge of a block or cushion. This will tip the pelvis forwards, ease pressure on the back, and shift the stretch to the intended target: the hamstrings.

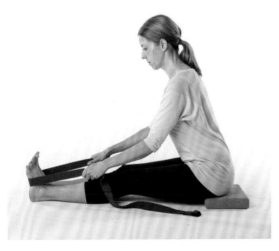

2 **Butterfly or Cross-Legged Pose** Sitting on a block or cushion elevates the hips which makes any wide-knee position, such as Butterfly or sitting cross-legged, a little more comfortable. Alternatively, place blocks or cushions under your knees.

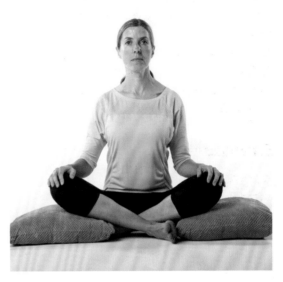

3 **Supporting your head** If your head tilts back when you lie down, rest it on a cushion or block to bring your head back in line with the spine. You are then in the correct position to proceed with any supine stretches without any neck strain.

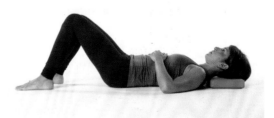

Stretching aid 3: foam brick

Foam bricks can be purchased from yoga or Pilates companies. These strong but lightweight rectangular brick-shaped blocks are worth sourcing especially if you have limited range of motion or suffer with lower backache. They 'bring the floor to your hands' rather than making you round your lower back to reach the floor in forward-bending stretches.

Here are three examples of foam block usage:

1 Wide-Legged Forward Bend If you lack the flexibility to bring the palms all the way to the floor, or want to protect an injured lower back, position your hands on two bricks at their tallest height.

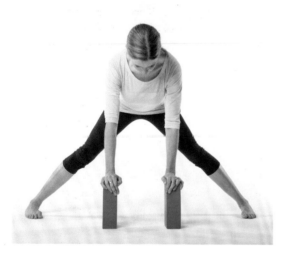

2 Low Lunge Positioning one brick either side of your hips where you can rest your hands enables you to stabilise the body and focus on dropping the hips deeper into the lunge.

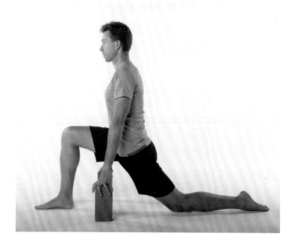

3 Lizard From all fours, step your left foot up to the outside of the left hand. Let your hips sink down. Either remain here with straight arms or slowly lower down onto the forearms. A brick under each forearm will raise the floor level and provide support for the upper body while you concentrate on stretching the hips and inner thighs. Repeat on the other side.

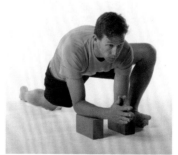

HOW TO USE THIS BOOK

If you are wondering how best to navigate this book, here is a quick guide. Decide what you'd like to achieve from the list below and turn to the relevant section. Here are a few examples:

- **A single stretch for a particular anatomical area or muscle, such as the hamstrings, trapezius or quadriceps.** The *Stretching by Anatomy* section offers a range of stretches for the neck and shoulders, wrists and hands, back and sides, hips and buttocks, upper legs, and lower legs and feet. They are grouped into standing, sitting and lying stretches and vary in intensity. Each anatomical section begins with a series of targeted warm-up moves to prepare for the deep, static stretches that follow.

- **A sequence of stretches for a particular anatomical area or muscle.** Each anatomical section in *Stretching By Anatomy* concludes with four 5-minute sequences so you can easily string individual stretches together for that body region.

- **Chair-based stretches for those lacking mobility or recovering from illness.** Most main stretches can be adapted to be performed while sitting on a chair. Turn to the *Stretches for Seniors* routine and the gentle *Total Body Flexibility* sequences. They are both found in the *Stretching Sequences* section.

- **A sequence for those who deem themselves 'stiff'.** Try the *Eight Stretches with a Strap* sequence (page 130) as it allows those lacking flexibility to access a range of stretches with the help of a cotton yoga strap, dressing gown belt or tie. The two Gentle *Total Body Flexibility* routines are also worth a look. The *Total Body Flexibility Gentle, Intermediate and Advanced* sequences repeat versions of the same stretches but the stretches increase in difficulty or intensity as you move up a level. This means that if you wish to improve your flexibility you can progress to the slightly deeper variation.

- **Advanced stretches for the more supple.** If you are naturally more supple or have been dedicating time to flexibility training perhaps for a sport that demands it, like a martial art, try the *Total Body Flexibility Advanced* sequences. At the end of each sport section in *Stretches by Sport*, there is also a 'Going Deeper' stretch for those wanting an advanced option.

- **Warm-up techniques and cool down stretches for football, running, cycling and 17 other sports.** The *Stretches by Sport* section offers six pre-sport warm-up moves and ten post-play stretches for 20 sports. The warm-up techniques raise the body temperature, improve mobility, reduce potential injuries and ingrain movement patterns. The static stretches restore muscle length, reduce recovery time, avoid injury and even aid performance. Picture a tennis player's wide lunge for the ball, a golfer coiling back in preparation to swing or a road cyclist dropping into an aerodynamic position.

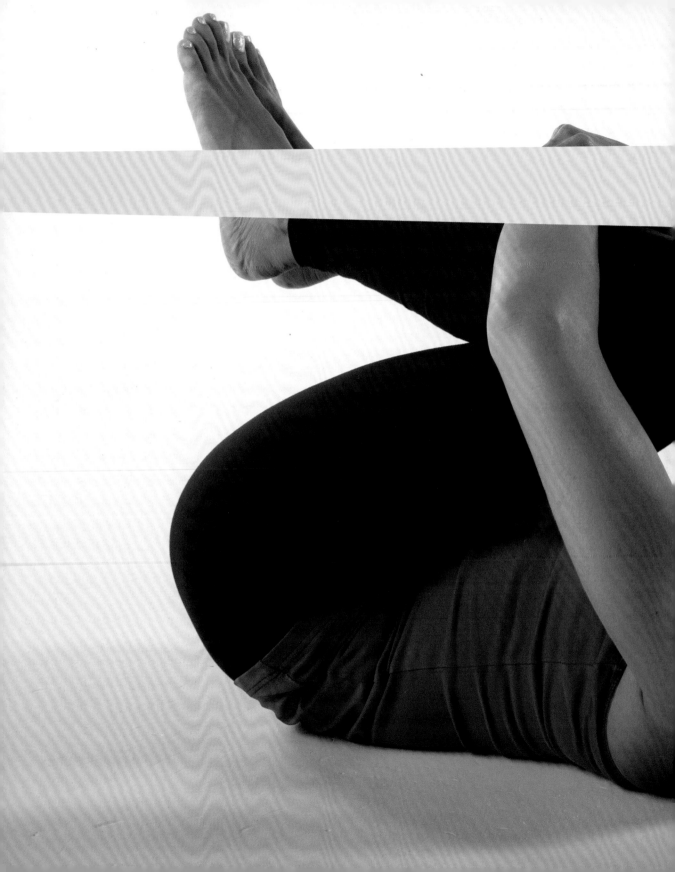

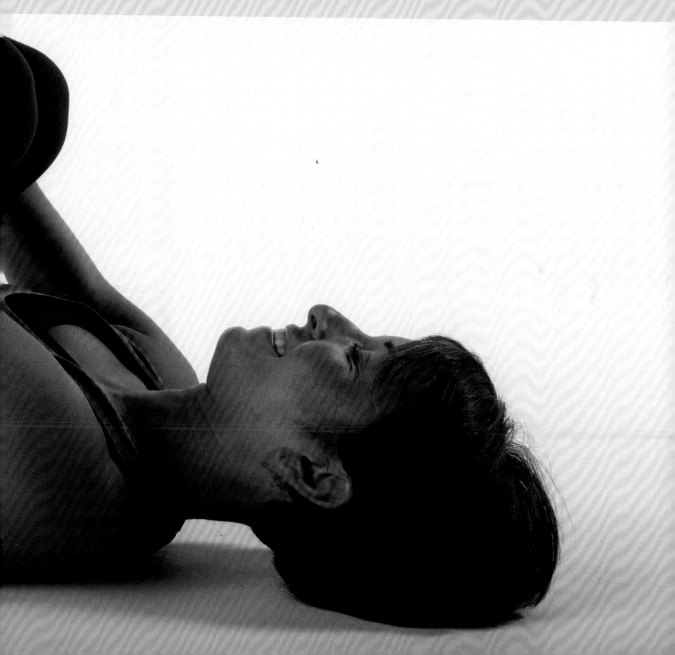

Stretching by Anatomy

Stretches for the Neck and Shoulders

Many of us have suffered with a stiff neck or shoulders at some point. This might be an overuse injury caused by playing a particular sport that involves repetitive head turning, such as swimming the front crawl, or being desk bound for long periods. Poor posture and stress can also trigger neck and shoulder tension. The good news is that neck and shoulder stretching is easy and convenient – as simple as rolling your shoulders in circles. It can be done at a desk or while commuting and often brings immediate relief.

Warm up the neck and shoulders first, then either select an individual stretch or two, or choose a sequence from the end of the chapter.

The Neck

WARMING UP

Repeat each technique x 4

HEAD ROLL

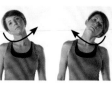

Make a continuous semi-circle movement with your head by first tipping your head to the right side by dropping your ear to your shoulder, looking down at your feet, then rolling your head around to the left shoulder. Move in slow motion. Don't tip your head back. Repeat in the other direction.

HEAD TURN

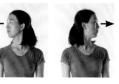

Rotate your head to the right, back to the centre and over to the left. Continue to turn your head from side to side. Move in slow motion.

HEAD NOD

Drop your head down, tucking the chin in towards the upper chest. Lift your head and look slightly up. Continue to nod your head slowly and smoothly.

HEAD TILT

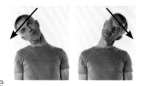

Look ahead. Tip your right ear down towards your right shoulder. Return to the centre. Tip your left ear down towards your left shoulder. Return to the centre. Continue to tilt your head from side to side slowly and smoothly.

Neck stretches

Hold each stretch for 20 seconds.

Take care not to overstretch the neck muscles as this may result in increased, rather than decreased, tightness. Progress slowly and gently and always stretch both sides of the neck muscles, even if one side is much tighter, to maintain muscle balance. When possible use just the weight of your head and let gravity do the work for you. The hands are used lightly in the 'assisted' neck stretches as a little extra weight or a light touch of the fingertips, but if this feels uncomfortable, do the version without the hands.

NECK EXTENSOR STRETCH

Stand or sit tall. Drop your head down, bringing your chin towards your chest. Let your head hang, allowing the weight of your head to do the stretching.

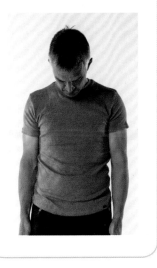

ASSISTED NECK EXTENSOR STRETCH

Stand or sit tall. Interlink your hands behind your head. Drop your head down bringing your chin towards your chest. Do not push your head further but let your elbows drop forwards so that the weight of your arms increases the stretch.

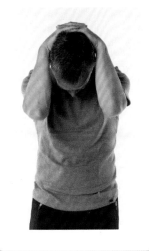

TRAPEZIUS STRETCH

Stand or sit tall. Drop your head down to look between your feet. Now turn your head slightly to the right to look at your right foot. Return your head to your starting position before repeating on the opposite side.

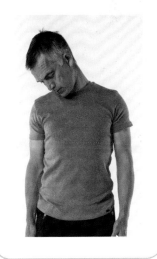

ASSISTED TRAPEZIUS STRETCH

Stand or sit tall. Drop your head down to look between your feet. Turn your head slightly to the right to look at your right foot. Raise your right arm up, place your right hand onto the top of your head and draw your head a little deeper into the stretch. Repeat on the other side.

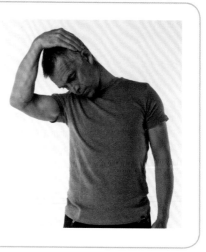

SIDE NECK STRETCH

Stand or sit tall with your arms by your side. Look forwards. Slowly lower your right ear to your right shoulder. To stretch deeper, press your left shoulder downwards. Repeat on the other side.

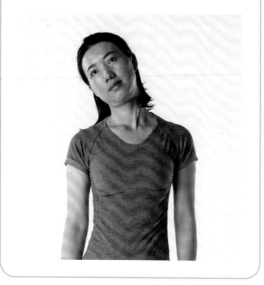

ASSISTED SIDE NECK STRETCH

Slowly lower your right ear to your right shoulder. Raise your right arm up and place your right palm onto the left side of your head. Gently draw your head a little further over to the right. Repeat on the other side.

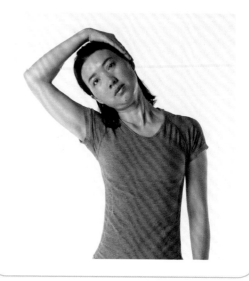

CLASPED HANDS NECK STRETCH

Take your hands behind your back. Interlink them and slide them around to the right side of your waist. Tip your head over to the right. Repeat on the other side.

ROTATING NECK STRETCH

Stand or sit tall. Keeping your shoulders straight, slowly rotate your head to the right bringing your chin towards your shoulder. Repeat on the other side.

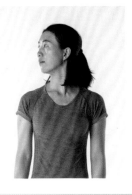

ASSISTED ROTATING NECK STRETCH

Repeat the Rotating Neck Stretch by turning your head to the right. Now bring your right fingertips to the left side of your chin and gently encourage the stretch.

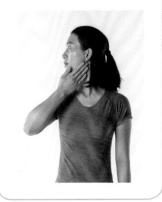

NECK FLEXOR STRETCH

Stand or sit tall. Raise your head as if looking at the ceiling. Keep your mouth closed and teeth together.

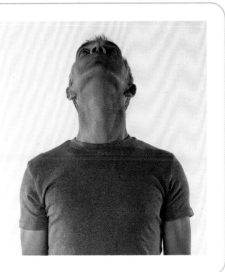

The Shoulders

In theory the ball and socket shoulder joint should be highly mobile, with your arm able to rotate 360 degrees, but the stiffening effects of older age, a sedentary job or even practising a sport, such as golf, climbing or tennis, can all gradually impact on shoulder mobility. This section provides a wide range of stretches for the shoulder girdle and surrounding areas including the chest muscles, which, if tight, can cause the back and shoulders to round, leading to slouching. Handpick one or two stretches if you want to target a particular muscle or work through a few sequences at the end of this chapter to maintain or improve overall shoulder health and mobility.

WARMING UP

Repeat each technique x 4

SWIMMING ARMS 1

Drop your fingertips onto your shoulders and 'swim' your arms by making alternate circles with your elbows. Roll your shoulders forwards first, then repeat in a backwards motion.

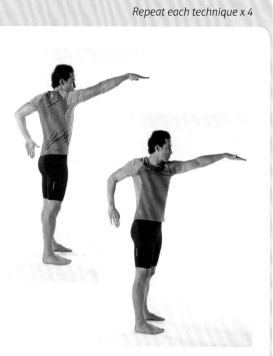

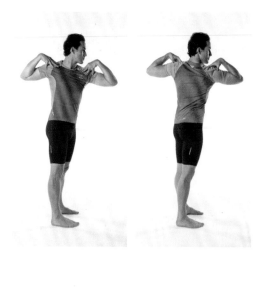

SWIMMING ARMS 2

'Swim' your arms, mimicking a front crawl movement. Allow the upper body to rotate as you reach forwards with alternate arms. Reverse the exercise by copying the backstroke movement.

WARMING UP (CONT.)

Repeat each technique x 4

ELBOW TOUCH

Drop your fingertips onto your shoulders. Sit or stand tall. Breathe in as you draw your elbows wide. Breathe out as you draw your elbows closer together in front of you. Touch them together if you can.

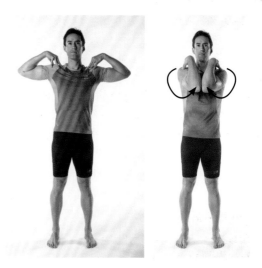

SHOULDER BLADE SQUEEZE

Position your arms in a 'W' shape. Draw your arms back and squeeze your shoulder blades together. Release and bring your forearms closer together, touching if you can.

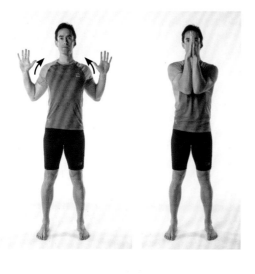

SHOULDER SHRUG

Lift your shoulders up towards your ears. Hold for a second. Now let them drop down.

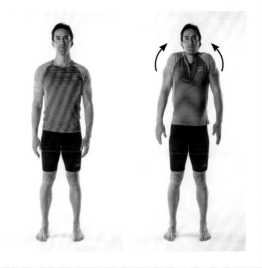

Shoulder stretches

Perform each stretch for 10-20 seconds.

Triceps stretch series

The following techniques target the triceps underneath your upper arm, but also the rotator muscles in your shoulder. If this is a tight area for you, proceed gently and slowly. Have a strap, belt or tie nearby as an aid.

TRICEPS STRETCH

Stand with your feet hip-distance apart. Reach up with your right arm and bend it so your hand drops behind your upper back. Use your left hand to gently draw your right elbow back. Repeat on the other side.

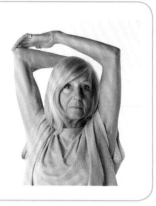

SHOULDER BLADE REACH STRETCH

Stand with your feet hip-distance apart. Take your left arm behind your back and slide your hand up the spine towards the middle of your shoulder blades. Repeat on the other side.

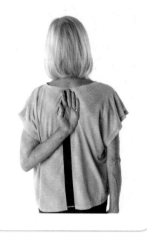

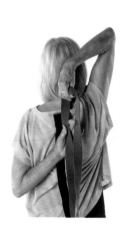

TRICEPS STRAP STRETCH

Lay a strap, belt or tie over your right shoulder. Repeat the Triceps Stretch with the right arm, but this time take your left arm behind your back and slide it up the spine. Use the strap to bridge the gap between your hands.

ADVANCED TRICEPS STRETCH

Reach up with your right arm and bend it so your hand drops behind your upper back. Taking your left hand behind your back, slide it up the spine and try to link your hands together. If you can't comfortably grip your hands together, then use a strap (see Triceps Strap Stretch). You may be able to link hands on one side, but not the other.

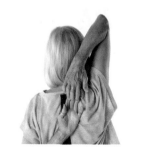

Back of shoulder stretch series

These stretches target the muscles in your upper back and posterior shoulders, such as the trapezius, the rhomboids and the posterior deltoid. If you have a niggling ache in the upper back, try these techniques, stopping at the stretch that suits your level of mobility. Those with broad shoulders or muscly biceps may struggle to perform the Advanced Arm Wrap Stretch, but this is purely due to physical build rather than insufficient flexibility so find a substitute stretch that suits your physique.

POSTERIOR SHOULDER STRETCH

Stand with your left arm straight and at chest height. Place your right arm behind your left elbow and draw the arm across your body. Do not rotate your torso. Repeat on the other side.

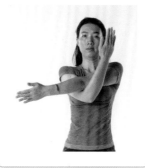

ARM WRAP STRETCH

Stand tall. Wrap your arms around your shoulders as if giving yourself a hug. Draw your shoulders away from your ears.

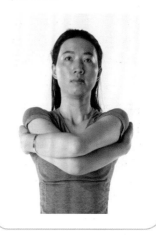

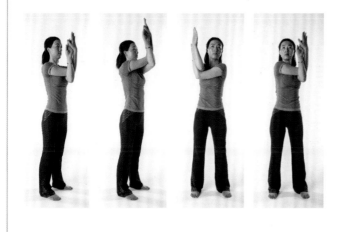

ADVANCED ARM WRAP

Stand tall and raise your arms to shoulder height. Wrap your right arm over your left so that your arms cross at the elbows. Now move your hands closer. Relax your shoulders away from your ears. Experiment with the following variations:

- Drawing your arms downwards
- Lifting your arms upwards
- Moving your arms to the right
- Moving your arms to the left

Unravel and repeat the stretch, crossing the left arm over the right.

Front of shoulder and chest stretch series

The shoulder muscles at the front of your body, such as the anterior deltoids, are covered here, but also the muscles of the chest or the 'pecs'. Why include pectoralis major and minor in a chapter on shoulders? Tight chest muscles have a direct effect on the shoulders by drawing them forwards or 'rounding' the upper back and shoulders. In yoga the following stretches would be known collectively as 'shoulder openers'. Proceed gently, stopping at the point of tension rather than discomfort or pain.

STRAP SHOULDER LOOSENER

Hold a strap or tie overhead with your hands wide apart and play with the following movements:

- Drop your hands forwards so the strap is in front of your chest.
- Lift the strap overhead so it is behind your head.
- Tilt to the left reaching your arms high.
- Tilt to the right reaching your arms high.

Repeat the whole sequence x 4.

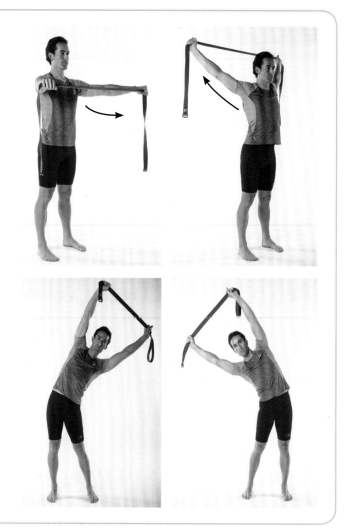

OVERHEAD STRAP STRETCH

Remain standing. Raise your strap, tie or belt overhead with your hands wide. Bend your arms until they form a 90-degree angle and draw your elbows back.

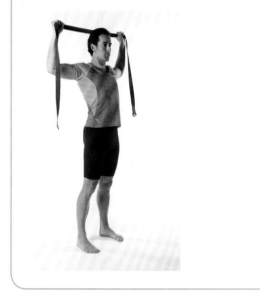

CHEST AND SHOULDER STRETCH

Take your arms behind your back and interlink your hands. Lift your chest, draw your shoulders back and raise your hands. Do not lean forward. Lift your hands higher to go deeper.

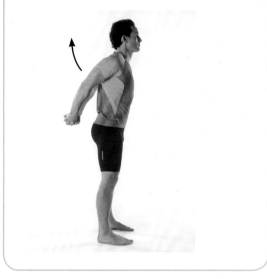

Shoulders Back! Stretching and Posture

Stretching can help prevent and correct poor posture caused partly by a combination of tight chest muscles and stretched or weak upper back muscles. Sit slouched for long periods and, over time, these tight chest muscles draw the shoulders forwards creating a rounded spine and sometimes a poking chin (picture a T-Rex side on and you get the idea). A combination of stretching and strengthening can correct bad posture by lengthening the chest muscles and strengthening the upper back. Try the Overhead Strap Stretch and the relaxing Rolled Mat Stretch (page 33). Also aim to sit or stand tall and draw your shoulders back as if flattening the shoulder blades whenever you remember. Strength exercises such as The Plank or the gym exercise Seated Row will reinforce the muscles of the upper back.

CHEST AND SHOULDER STRAP STRETCH

Repeat the Chest and Shoulder Stretch, holding a strap between your hands, but this time bend your knees, tip forwards from the hips, drop your head and lift your hands off the lower back. Remain here for 20-30 seconds, letting the weight of your arms drop forwards. To exit, drop the strap to your lower back, bend your knees deeply and rise up to a standing position.

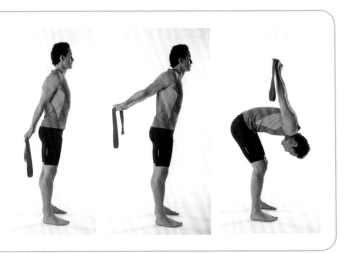

PARTNER CHEST AND SHOULDER STRETCHES

Try the following shoulder and chest stretches with a partner. Having someone assist the stretch means you can go deeper than stretching solo. Just ensure that you proceed with caution by maintaining communication with your partner and stopping the stretch at the initial point of tension or the 'edge' of the stretch.

1 Stand tall with your partner behind you. Raise both arms up horizontally. Ask your partner to hold your hands or wrists and gently draw your arms backwards while you maintain a straight back. Turn your palms to face outwards. Stop when you feel the point of tension.

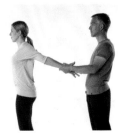

2 Sit on a chair. Clasp your hands behind your head and relax your shoulders. Ask your partner to stand behind you, hold your elbows and gently draw your arms back.

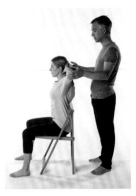

3 Remain seated. Drop your fingertips on to the tops of your shoulders. Ask your partner to stand behind you, hold your elbows and gently draw your arms back.

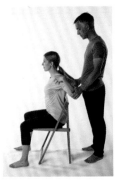

THE RACK

Sit on the floor with your legs straight. Take your hands behind your back and press them into the mat. Lift your chest, but keep your chin tucked in. Squeeze your shoulder blades together. Position your hands closer together or further back from your body to go deeper. Note: this is a deep stretch for your shoulders so avoid it or only do the first part of the stretch if you have an injury.

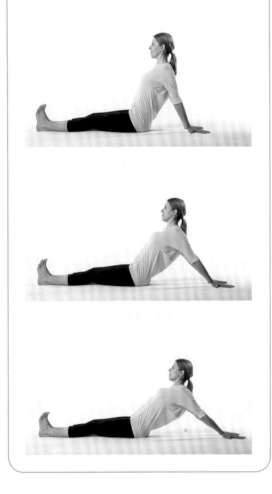

'PASSIVE' STRETCHING: WORKING WITH GRAVITY

The term 'passive' stretching denotes techniques that simply let gravity do the work. The idea is to get comfortable, remain still, breathe deeply through the nose, and let the legs or arms relax. Hold a little longer than a normal stretch – up to 1 or 2 minutes – but exit slowly and carefully. The Rolled Mat Stretch is an example of a passive stretch and is particularly useful for people who spend time with a flexed spine, such as desk workers, drivers, as well as cyclists. Passive stretching is also a useful wind-down technique for people who find it hard to sleep as, when it's combined with slow breathing, it's half stretch and half relaxation technique.

ROLLED MAT STRETCH

You will need a yoga mat or similar long exercise mat for this stretch. Roll it up tightly. Sit on the front edge of the mat and lower yourself down to lying. Ensure that your head and hips are on the mat. Bend your legs and place your feet on the floor. Bend your arms into a right angle position. Remain here for 1-3 minutes relaxing the arms as much as possible.

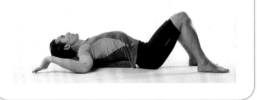

Five-minute stretch sequences

String together some stretches into five-minute routines for the neck and shoulder region.

Neck sequence 1

1. HEAD NOD

Drop your head down tucking the chin in towards your upper chest. Lift your head and look slightly up. Continue to nod your head slowly and smoothly. *Repeat x 4.*

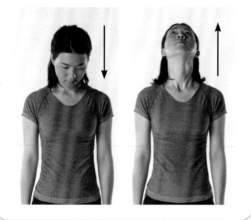

2. HEAD TILT

Look ahead. Tip your right ear down towards your right shoulder. Return to the centre. Tip your left ear down towards your left shoulder. Return to the centre. Continue to tilt your head from side to side slowly and smoothly. *Repeat x 4.*

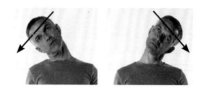

3. ASSISTED NECK EXTENSOR STRETCH

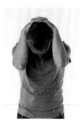

Stand or sit tall. Interlink your hands behind your head. Drop your head down, bringing your chin towards your chest. Do not push your head further down, but let your elbows drop forward so that the weight of your arms increases the stretch.

DOORFRAME SHOULDER STRETCH

A doorway is the perfect space to stretch the front of your shoulders and your chest muscles. Standing tall in the middle of the doorway, raise your arms out sideways at chest height, place your palms on the wall either side of the doorframe, and lean your chest into the space. Try repeating the above with your arms in a higher V-shaped position.

4. ASSISTED TRAPEZIUS STRETCH

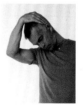

Stand or sit tall. Drop your head down to look between your feet. Turn your head slightly to the right to look at your right foot. Raise your right arm up, place your right hand onto the top of your head and draw your head a little deeper into the stretch. Repeat on the other side.

Neck sequence 2

1. HEAD ROLL

Make a continuous semi-circle movement with your head by first tipping your head to the right side by dropping your ear to your shoulder, looking down at your feet, then rolling your head around to the left shoulder. Move in slow motion. Don't tip your head back. Repeat in the other direction. *Repeat x 4.*

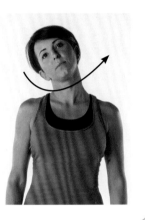

2. HEAD TURN

Rotate your head to the right, back to the centre and over to the left. Continue to turn your head from side to side. Move in slow motion. *Repeat x 4.*

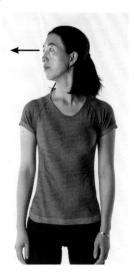

3. ASSISTED ROTATING NECK STRETCH

Stand or sit tall. Keeping your shoulders straight, slowly rotate your head to the right bringing your chin towards your shoulder. Now bring your right fingertips to the left side of the chin and gently encourage the stretch. *Hold for 10 seconds on each side.*

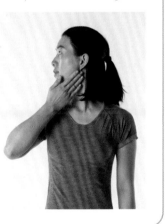

4. NECK FLEXOR STRETCH

Stand tall. Raise your head as if looking to the ceiling. Keep your mouth closed and teeth together. *Hold for 10 seconds.*

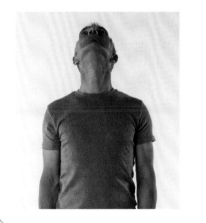

Shoulder sequence 1

1. SWIMMING ARMS 1

Drop your fingertips onto your shoulders and 'swim' your arms by making alternate circles with your elbows. Roll your shoulders first forwards, then in a backwards motion. *Repeat x 6.*

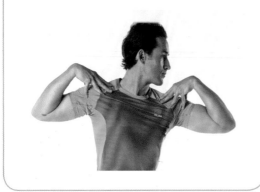

2. POSTERIOR SHOULDER STRETCH

Stand with your left arm straight and at chest height. Place your right arm behind your left elbow and draw your arm across your body. Do not rotate the torso. *Hold for 10-20 seconds.*

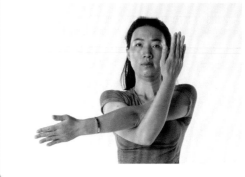

3. TRICEPS STRETCH

Stand with your feet hip-width apart. Reach up with your right arm and bend it so your hand drops behind your upper back. Use your left hand to gently draw your right elbow back. *Hold for 10-20 seconds.*

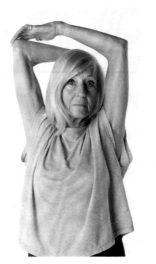

4. SHOULDER STRETCH

Take your arms behind your back and interlink your hands. Lift your chest, draw your shoulders back and raise your hands. To go deeper, bring the palms of your hands together while your hands are clasped. *Hold for 10-20 seconds.*

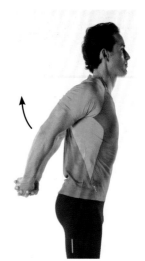

Shoulder sequence 2

1. SHOULDER SHRUG

Lift your shoulders up towards your ears. Hold for a second. Now let them drop down. *Repeat x 4.*

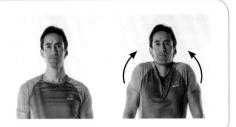

2. STRAP SHOULDER LOOSENER

Hold a strap or tie overhead with your hands wide apart. Drop your hands forwards so the strap is in front of your chest, then lift the strap overhead so it is behind your head. *Repeat x 4.*

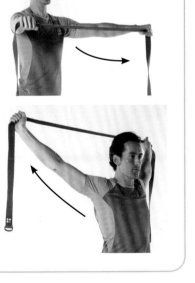

3. OVERHEAD STRAP STRETCH

Remain standing. Raise your strap, tie or belt overhead with your hands wide. Bend your arms until they form a 90-degree angle and draw your elbows back. *Hold for 20 seconds.*

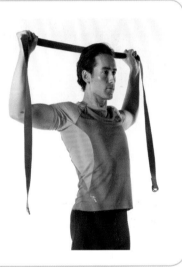

4. ARM WRAP STRETCH

Stand tall. Wrap your arms around your shoulders as if giving yourself a hug. Draw your shoulders away from your ears. *Hold for 10 seconds.*

Stretches for the Wrists and Hands

A little diligent stretching of the delicate hand and wrist muscles is wise if you spend long hours at a keyboard to prevent conditions such as Repetitive Strain Injury. Sportspeople, such as squash or tennis players, can use these stretches to ensure their hands, wrists and forearms can withstand the repeated impact of hitting the ball. Don't overstretch by applying pressure too quickly.

Wrists and Hands

This section contains both stand-alone stretches and ready-made sequences for the delicate muscles of the wrists and hands. It is aimed at anyone wanting to ease stiffness or maintain flexibility in this region. Regular gentle stretching may also help prevent common wrist/hand problems such as Repetitive Strain Injury (RSI). Please note: if you already have inflammation in the wrists or hands stretching may be harmful; see a medical professional for advice.

WARMING UP

WRIST ROLL
Make fists with both hands and rotate them slowly.

SQUEEZE AND SPREAD
Squeeze your hands into fists, tucking the thumb in and hold for five seconds. Now spread your hands wide and hold for five seconds. *Repeat x 4.*

WRIST AND HAND WARMER
Interlace your fingers, palms down and chest-height. Pull your

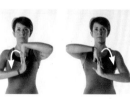

hands slightly apart as if your fingers were stuck together. Alternate between flexing and extending (bending and drawing back) your wrists.

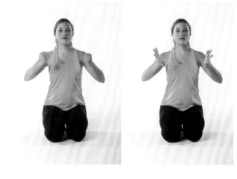

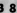

Body part stretches

STANDING WRIST EXTENSOR STRETCH

Hold your right arm out straight. Grasp your right fingers and draw them back towards your palm.

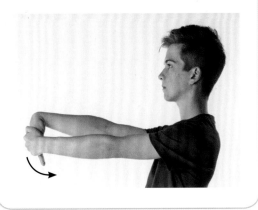

STANDING WRIST FLEXOR STRETCH

Hold your right arm out straight. Lift your fingers and draw them back towards your body.

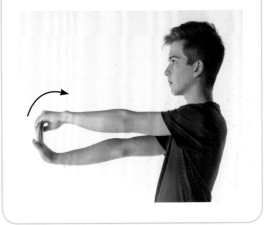

KNEELING WRIST FLEXOR STRETCH

From a kneeling position, lean forwards and gently prepare to place your palms on the floor in front of you with the fingers pointing back to your knees. Proceed to lay more of the palms onto the floor if this feels comfortable.

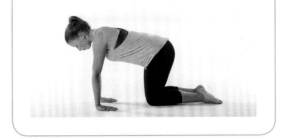

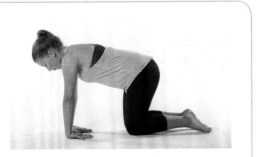

KNEELING WRIST EXTENSOR STRETCH

From a kneeling position, lean forwards and gently position the backs of your hands on the floor with the fingers pointing back to your knees. Begin by pressing the fingertips into the floor and only lay more of the back of your hands on the floor if this feels comfortable.

Repetitive Strain Injury

Repetitive Strain Injury, or RSI, is a general term to describe the pain felt in muscles, nerves and tendons caused by repetitive movement or overuse. It is often triggered by large amounts of time spent typing, and symptoms include tingling or numbness, cramp, stiffness or pain. If you are already experiencing symptoms of RSI, see your doctor or physiotherapist first as some stretches can do more harm than good. But if you spend large amounts of time at a keyboard, the stretches in this chapter are a good preventative measure to avoid suffering with what can be a frustrating condition. Try The Prayer Stretch series once or twice a day. Setting up your workplace correctly, strengthening exercises and taking regular breaks from the keyboard are also recommended steps to take.

THE PRAYER STRETCH SERIES

1 Place your palms together at chest height in a prayer position. Keeping your palms connected, slowly lower your hands until your arms reach a 90-degree position. Hold each step for 10 seconds.

2 Tip your hands to the left.

3 Tip your hands to the right.

4 Move your hands outwards so your fingers are pointing away from you.

5 Place the backs of your hands together with your fingers pointed down.

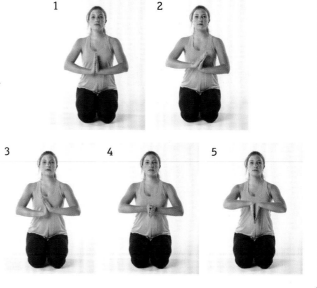

FINGER STRETCH

Spread your fingers wide. Gently draw back each finger one by one, holding for a few seconds.

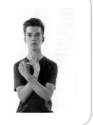

THUMBS UP

Make a 'thumbs up' position by curling your fingers into your palm with your thumb sticking up and gently draw your thumb back.

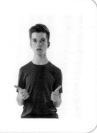

Five-minute stretch sequences

String together some stretches into five-minute routines for the forearms, wrists and hands.

Wrists and hands sequence 1

1. WRIST ROLL

Make fists with both hands and rotate them slowly. *Repeat x 4.*

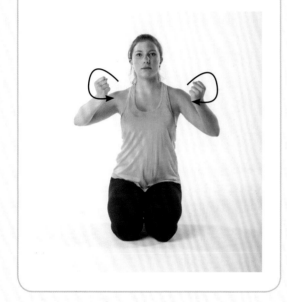

2. SQUEEZE AND SPREAD

Squeeze your hands into fists tucking the thumb in and hold for five seconds. Now spread your hands wide and hold for five seconds. *Repeat x 4.*

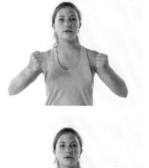

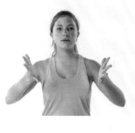

3. FINGER STRETCHING

Spread your fingers wide. Gently draw back each finger one by one. *Hold for 3-4 seconds.*

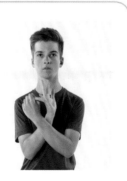

4. THUMBS UP

Make a 'thumbs up' position by curling your fingers into your palm with your thumb sticking up and gently draw your thumb back. *Hold for 5 seconds.*

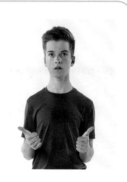

Wrists and hands sequence 2

1. STANDING WRIST EXTENSOR STRETCH

Hold your right arm out straight. Grasp your right fingers and draw them back towards your palm. *Hold for 10 seconds.*

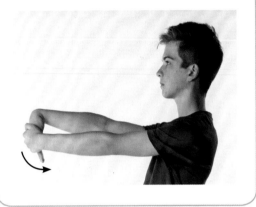

2. STANDING WRIST FLEXOR STRETCH

Hold your right arm out straight. Lift your fingers and draw them back towards your body. *Hold for 10 seconds.*

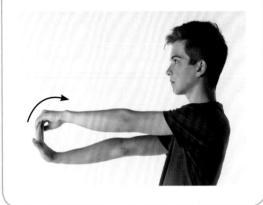

3. PRAYER STRETCH 2

Place your palms together at chest height in a prayer position. Tip your hands to the left. *Hold for 10 seconds.*

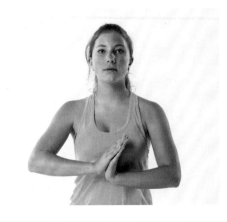

4. PRAYER STRETCH 3

Place your palms together at chest height in a prayer position. Tip your hands to the right. *Hold for 10 seconds.*

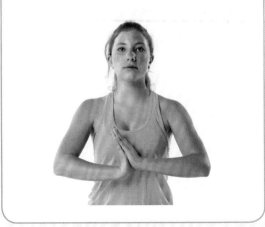

Wrists and hands sequence 3

1. WRIST ROLL

Make fists with both hands and rotate them slowly. *Repeat x 4.*

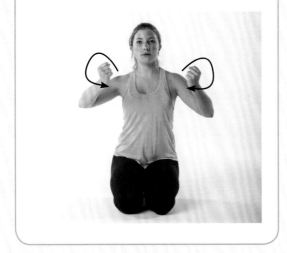

2. FINGER STRETCHING

Spread your fingers wide. Gently draw back each finger one by one. *Hold for 3-4 seconds.*

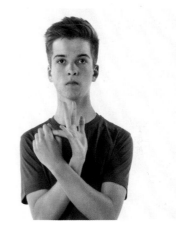

3. WRIST FLEXOR STRETCH KNEELING

From a kneeling position, gently place your palms on the floor with the fingers pointing back to your knees. Begin by pressing the fingertips onto the floor and only lay more of your palm down if this feels comfortable. *Hold for 10 seconds.*

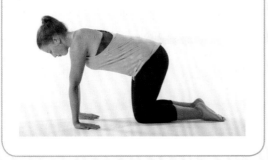

4. WRIST EXTENSOR STRETCH KNEELING

From a kneeling position, gently place the backs of your hands on the floor, fingers pointing to your knees. Continue by laying more of the back of your hand onto the floor if this feels comfortable. *Hold for 10 seconds.*

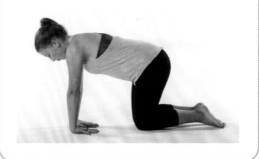

Stretches for the Back and Sides

Aching lower back? Providing that this is a mild, muscular ache and nothing more serious (always see a doctor or physiotherapist if you are unsure), regular, gentle stretching can keep the back healthy, supple and injury free. For easy navigation this chapter groups back stretching techniques both into physical positions (lying, all fours, chair or standing) as well as anatomical areas (lower, mid and upper back) if you need to target a more specific region. It ends with a selection of five-minute whole back sequences that string the individual stretches into short routines. These may be practised individually or joined together to create a comprehensive 20-minute routine that will maintain whole back mobility.

The Back and Sides

WARMING UP   *Repeat each technique x 4*

STANDING TWIST

Starting in a standing position, bend your knees and relax your arms by your sides. Twist your upper body to the left and let the arms swing around. Return to the centre and twist to the right.

MID-BACK WARM-UP

Start in a standing position with a small bend in your knees. Move your arms into a 90-degree position. Keep your hips and legs still and twist your upper body slowly and gently from side to side.

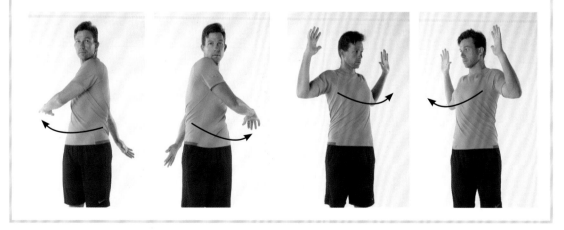

Standing back and side stretches

FULL BODY STRETCH

Stand with your feet hip-width apart. Sweep your arms up overhead and interlink your fingers. Press your palms towards the ceiling and remain here. Lift your arms up, but relax your shoulders.

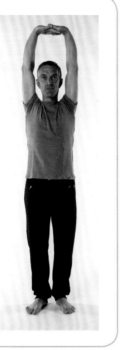

STANDING BACK BEND

Stand with your feet hip-width apart. Place your hands on your lower back, fingers pointing downwards. Continue looking forward or slightly down. Lean back. Push your hips forward. Draw your elbows together.

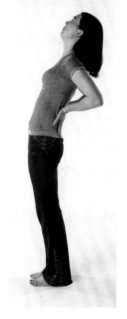

STANDING SIDE BEND

Stand with your feet hip-width apart. Sweep your arms up overhead and interlink your fingers. Then simply lean to the side aiming not to tip forwards or backwards. To go deeper, try clasping the top wrist and bend sideways further. Repeat on the other side.

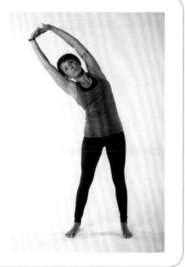

THE TRIANGLE

Step your feet wide with your feet facing forward. Turn your right foot out 90 degrees and your left foot in 45 degrees. Raise your arms up to shoulder height. Tip your upper body to the right. Lightly rest your right hand on your leg. Either reach your left arm up or reach it over by your left ear to perform the more advanced version. Repeat on the other side.

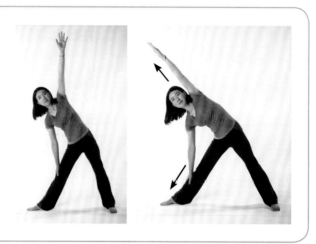

SLOW ROLL DOWN

Stand with a slight bend in your knees. Drop your head down, lean a little forward and let your arms dangle. Start to roll down in slow motion by letting your upper back, then mid back, round. Roll slowly back up. *Note: Don't roll too far if you have problems with your lower back.*

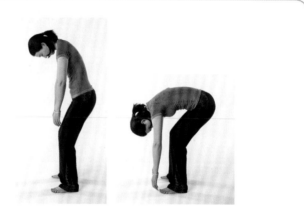

Decompressing the Back

If the whole back just feels tight and you can't pinpoint a specific area to stretch, these techniques will provide a deeply satisfying feeling of decompression and muscular release for both the back and shoulders. This can be as simple as clasping the top of a doorframe and bending your knees to lengthen the muscles of the back while keeping your feet on the floor.

Or try the 90-degree Chair Stretch on page 56, placing your hands on the back of a chair and tipping your body into a 90-degree position. You can deepen the intensity of the back stretch by pressing your hands on to the chair and moving your hips back in the opposite direction. Kitchen counters are also generally at a good height to try this back decompressing stretch on.

The all fours series

CAT STRETCH

Start on all fours. As you inhale, lift your head and hips, allowing the mid back to dip. As you exhale, tuck the chin in and the hips under, allowing the back to round. *Repeat x 4.*

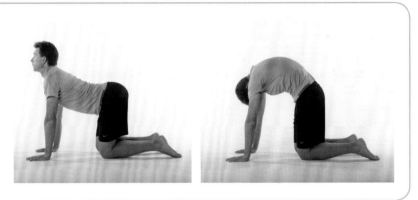

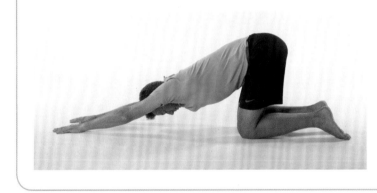

PUPPY DOG STRETCH

Start on all fours, keeping your knees positioned under your hips. Walk your hands forwards until your head and chest lower towards the floor. To exit, draw your abdomen in and slowly walk your hands back.

KNEELING BACK STRETCH

From all fours, sit back on your heels. Straighten your arms and reach your hands in front of you. Spread your fingers and press down. Pull back, away from your hands, for a deeper stretch.

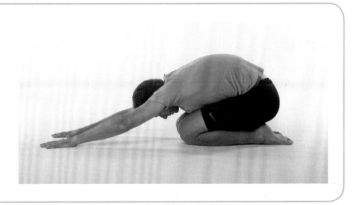

KNEELING BACK STRETCH WITH HOOKED THUMBS

From all fours, sit back on your heels. Reach your hands in front of you and bring them close together. Spread your fingers and press down. Hook your thumbs together. Draw your hips away in the opposite direction.

KNEELING SIDE STRETCH

From all fours, sit back on your heels with your hands stretched out together in front of you, walk your hands over to the right. Press your palms into the floor. Walk your hands over to the left and press your palms into the floor.

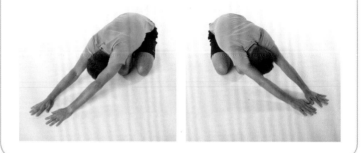

CHILD'S POSE

From all fours, lower yourself slowly down to sit on your heels. Rest your forehead on the floor and relax your arms by your sides. If your forehead does not reach the floor, place some foam blocks or cushions under your forehead.

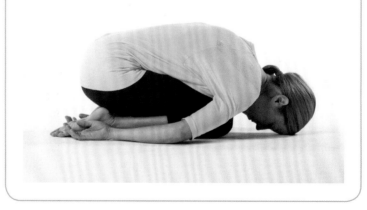

The twist series

Gentle rotation of the trunk is a great way to loosen tight back muscles. Just ensure with the sitting twist techniques that you don't allow the more mobile lower back and neck to do all the rotation. When teaching seated spinal twists, I encourage students to divide the rotation into three parts: first, turn from the lower back and stop; then, turn from the middle back and shoulders and stop; and finally, rotate your head as far as is comfortable.

BASIC SEATED TWIST

Sit with your legs out straight. Bend your left leg and step it over your right. Wrap your right arm around your leg and hug your leg into your body. Drop your left fingertips onto the floor behind your back and begin to rotate the torso to the left in stages: lower back, mid back and shoulders, and head. Repeat on the other side.

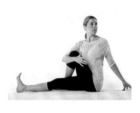

BASIC LYING TWIST

Lie on your back. Bend both legs, placing your feet flat on the floor. Stretch your arms out at shoulder height, palms facing upwards. Lower both legs down to the floor on the left side and relax them. Repeat on the other side.

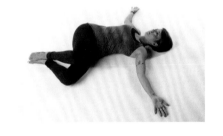

ADVANCED LYING TWIST 1

Lie on your back. Loop a strap around your right foot. Hold onto both parts of the strap with your left hand and slowly draw your leg across your body to the left. Repeat on the other side.

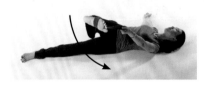

ADVANCED LYING TWIST 2

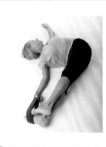

Lie on your back. Bend both legs, placing your feet flat on the floor. Stretch your arms out shoulder-height, palms facing upwards. Lower both legs down to the floor on the right side. Hold onto your toes with your right hand or loop a strap around the soles of your feet and hold the strap, and straighten your legs. Repeat on the other side.

TARGETING THE UPPER BACK

This section hones in on the muscles around the upper back which link into the neck and shoulders. If you are prone to tight muscles or injury in this area, do consult the earlier section Stretching for the Neck and Shoulders, because, as much as I would like to compartmentalise the body into neat categories, the muscles of the upper back, neck and shoulders are hard to isolate. The following sequence of stretches provides an overall stretch for the whole upper back region.

STANDING UPPER BACK ROUNDER

Stand with your feet hip-width apart. Round your upper back and tuck your chin in. Reach both arms forwards and interlock your fingers and turn your palms away to face outwards.

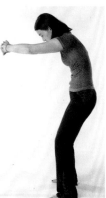

ASSISTED TRAPEZIUS STRETCH

Drop your head and tip it slightly to the right. Raise your right arm up, place your right hand onto the top of your head. Gently draw your head a little deeper into the stretch. Repeat on the other side.

ARM WRAP STRETCH

Stand tall. Wrap your arms around your shoulders as if giving yourself a hug. Draw your shoulders away from your ears.

ADVANCED ARM WRAP STRETCH

Wrap your left arm over your right to cross your arms. Now bring your palms closer together or touching. Draw your shoulders away from your ears. Unravel and repeat on the other side.

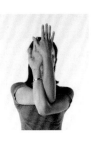

Shoulder Blade Squeezing

A simple way to rinse tension out of the upper back muscles is to first draw the shoulder blades down, away from your ears, then squeeze them a bit closer together. Squeeze your shoulder blades for a few seconds, then release and repeat x 4.

I find it helps to imagine you have someone standing behind you with their palms pressed to your shoulder blades. Visualise them sliding your shoulder blades down your back and then moving your shoulder blades closer together. This exercise can be done standing, sitting or on all fours and is a great but simple technique for improving posture.

TARGETING THE MID BACK

Compared to the lower back and neck, the mid-back – known as the thoracic spine – is often less mobile. Many people are stiff in this thoracic region. Here are some techniques that focus on the mid back.

ROUNDED BACK STRETCH

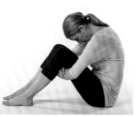

Sit with your legs bent and feet on the floor. Clasp your hands around the back of your thighs. Round your back, let your head drop down and lean back. *Hold for 30-60 seconds.*

ALL FOURS MID-BACK TWIST

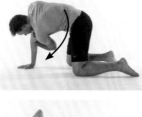

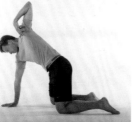

Start on all fours with your knees wide apart and your hands under your shoulders. Place your left fingertips on your left shoulder. Stay looking down. As you inhale, point the left elbow up to the ceiling. As you exhale, point the left elbow under the right armpit. *Repeat on the other side.*

LYING MID-BACK LOOSENER

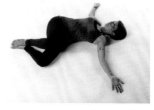

Lie on your back. Bend both legs, placing your feet flat on the floor. Stretch your arms out at shoulder height, palms facing upwards. Lower both legs down to the floor on your left side. Lift your right arm off the floor, roll onto your left side and lay your right palm on top of your left. Sweep your right arm back again to return to the start position. Move in slow motion. Repeat on the other side. *Repeat x 4.*

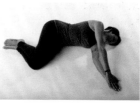

DEEP DOUBLE LEG HUG

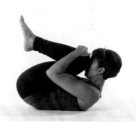

Lie on your back and hug both legs into your abdomen. Now draw your legs in closer and raise your head up towards your knees as if tucking yourself into a tight ball. Rock a little from side to side across the mid back. *Hold for 20 seconds.*

The Stiff Mid-Back in Sport

Thoracic or mid-back stretches are particularly beneficial both for cyclists and people who are required to rotate or twist their torsos to hit a ball, such as golfers or tennis players. Road cyclists spend hours locked in a rounded or flexed-back position, meaning the muscles of their mid back are constantly contracted. A stiff mid back also prevents the more aerodynamic, flatter-backed posture that riders desire. Golfers require a good level of flexibility in the mid-back region to facilitate the coiling back movement as they prepare to release the club in the golf swing. A stiff mid back not only affects comfort levels, performance or posture, but places greater pressure on the lower back to curve or twist. For targeted warm-up and cool down stretches for both sports, turn to *Stretching for Sport* (page 164).

Strengthening the Lower Back

To truly protect the lower back against aches or injury a combination of both muscle lengthening *and* strengthening is the key. A supple but strong back is a healthy back. This does not necessarily mean heading to the gym to lift dumbbells (unless under the watchful eye of a personal trainer), but using your own body weight as resistance. Perform the Cobra (see page 54) by lying face down with your forehead resting on the mat and arms by your sides, palms facing downwards and play with the following variations:

1 Rest your upper body on the floor. Slowly raise and lower alternate legs off the floor keeping your hips still and level. *Repeat x 6.*

2 Rest your legs on the floor and lift your upper body and arms a few inches off. *Hold for 10 seconds.*

3 Lift the feet and the upper body a few inches off the mat. *Hold for 10 seconds.*

4 Sit back in Child's Pose (page 48). *Hold for 20-30 seconds.*

TARGETING THE LOWER BACK

For niggling lower backache sometimes all that is required is a few simple movements to unlock muscular tension, such as lying on your back and drawing the legs into your chest. These stretches can be done first thing in the morning, even while still in bed, to loosen up the lower back. Experiment with a few of the techniques outlined below for some relief from discomfort or simply to keep the lower back supple and mobile. I have included stretches for both your hip flexors, located at the top of the thighs, and your hamstrings as lack of flexibility in both these areas can contribute to lower backache. Remember, if you are experiencing lower back pain rather than a muscular ache, consult a medical professional before attempting any stretching.

SINGLE LEG HUG

Lie on your back and hug your right leg in towards your chest. Keep your left leg straight and press the back of your left knee into the floor. Repeat on the other side. *Hold for 20 seconds.*

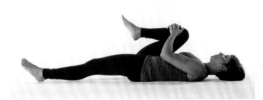

DOUBLE LEG HUG

Lie on your back and hug both legs into your abdomen. Rock a little from side to side across the lower back. *Hold for 20 seconds.*

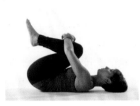

PELVIC TILTS

Lie on your back with your legs bent and feet on the floor. Have your arms by your sides. Keep your hips on the floor throughout. First, tilt your pelvis up by pressing your lower back into the

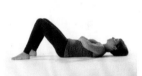

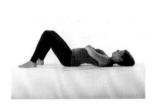

floor. Now tilt your pelvis back by lifting your belly button up to the ceiling. *Repeat x 4.*

BASIC LYING TWIST

Lie on your back. Bend both legs and place your feet flat on the floor. Stretch your arms out at shoulder height, palms facing upwards. Lower both legs down to the floor on the left side and relax them.

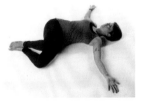

Warning: Watch your Back

Prone stretches where you lie on your front and push up, such as the Cobra, can aggravate the lower back muscles, so if this is a sensitive area for you, try a very low Cobra where you rise just an inch off the floor. Drop and lower the moment you have a feeling of compression in the lower back. Also, sit back in Child's Pose or Kneeling Back Stretch (see page 47) afterwards.

SPHINX

Lie down on your front positioning your elbows directly under your shoulders with the forearms parallel. Draw your shoulder blades slightly closer together.

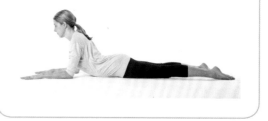

SNAKE

Lie on your front with your hands interlocked behind your back. Lift your upper body and legs a little off the floor. Tuck your chin in so you are looking down, not forwards.

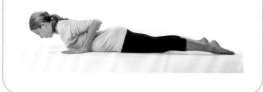

STRIKING COBRA

Lie on your front with your hands under your shoulders. Press into your hands and slowly raise your upper body off the ground until the arms are almost straight. Keep your hips on the floor. Lower down and sit back on your heels.

COBRA

Lie on your front with your hands under your shoulders. Press into your hands and slowly lift your upper body off the ground. Lower down and sit back on your heels.

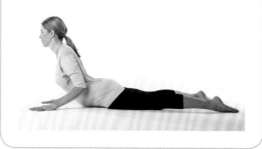

Lunging to Ease Lower Backache

Sometimes the best stretch to prevent lower backache does not actually involve the back muscles. The iliopsoas muscle or 'hip flexors', which can be felt at the top and front of the thigh, should be targeted too. Short or tight hip flexors can affect the alignment of the pelvis and put pressure on the vertebral discs. The best stretch for the hip flexors is the Low Lunge outlined below, so do practise the stretch if you are susceptible to lower back pain especially if your job involves plenty of time spent sitting.

LOW LUNGE

Lower down to all fours. Step your right foot up in between your hands and raise your upper body. Push your hips forward. Slowly lower into the lunge. Repeat on the other side.

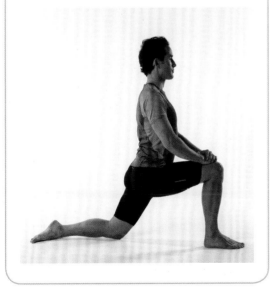

Tight Hamstrings and Lower Backache

It is also worth including a simple stretch for your hamstrings when stretching your lower back as a lack of flexibility in the hamstrings can place pressure on this region. The best way to stretch your hamstrings without aggravating the lower back is to do the Strap Hamstring Stretch. If the hamstrings feel very tight, bend your upper leg and don't try to straighten or lock your lower leg. Hold the stretch for 30-60 seconds and repeat on the other side. Hamstrings take diligent stretching, but try to perform this technique at least three times a week, or more frequently if possible.

STRAP HAMSTRING STRETCH

Lie on your back, looping a strap, belt or tie around the sole of the left foot. Bend the right leg and place the foot on the floor, especially if your hamstrings are tight. Straighten the left leg up towards the ceiling or keep it a little bent. Repeat on the other side.

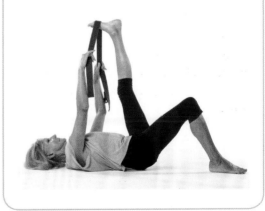

Chair stretch series

The following techniques would suit both older people and those with desk-based jobs who tend to suffer with stiffness, particularly in the lower back and upper back and shoulder region. For more whole body chair sequences turn to The Desk Worker (page 114) and Stretching for Seniors (page 128) routines.

CHAIR CAT STRETCH

Sit on a chair. Rest your hands lightly on your thighs. As you inhale, arch your back and look upwards a little. As you exhale, round your back and tuck your pelvis and chin in.

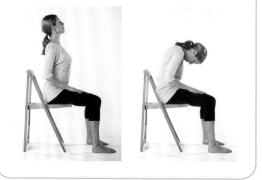

90-DEGREE CHAIR STRETCH

Stand behind a chair and place your hands on the top of the chair back, shoulder-width apart. Walk backwards until you fold into a 90-degree position. Move your head in line with your spine. To exit, draw your abdomen inwards, bend your knees and rise up to standing.

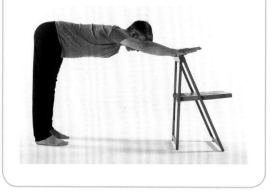

CHAIR SHOULDER BLADE SQUEEZE

Sitting on a chair, position your arms in a 'W' shape with your elbows close to your sides. Draw your arms back and squeeze your shoulder blades together. Hold for a few seconds, then release. *Repeat x 4.*

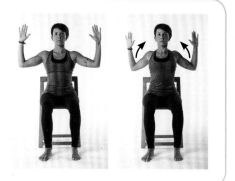

CHAIR BACK STRETCH

Sitting on a chair, sweep your arms up overhead and interlink your fingers. Press your palms towards the ceiling and hold this position, drawing your shoulders downwards.

CHAIR SIDE BEND

Sitting on a chair, sweep your right arm up overhead. Now simply lean to the side aiming not to tip forwards or backwards. To go deeper, try clasping the top wrist and side bending further.

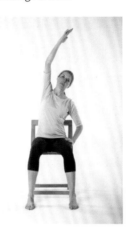

CHAIR FORWARD BEND

Sitting on a chair, round the back and let your head drop downwards. If the back feels very stiff, rest your hands on your thighs or lean further forwards until your hands touch the floor.

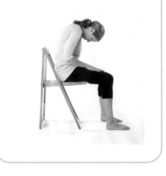

CHAIR BACK BEND

Sitting on a chair, place your hands on your thighs and draw your elbows closer. Lift your elbows up a little to feel a slight arch in the back.

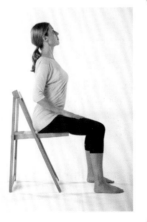

CHAIR TWIST

Sit tall on a chair. Hold onto the right side of your chair and rotate your torso to the right in sections: lower back, mid back and shoulders, and finally turn your head. Repeat on the other side.

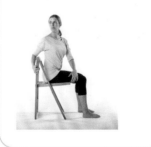

THE BACK: STRETCH OR RELAX?

Sometimes the answer is not an active stretch but a passive muscular release. We can 'switch off' contracted back muscles by resting or relaxing the back in various poses, such as lying on your back with your legs elevated on a chair or lying face down on the edge of a bed.

Try the following:

- **Chair Back Relaxer** Lie on your back with your legs bent and lower legs and feet resting on the seat of a chair. Your lower back should rest comfortably on the floor.
- **Bed Back Relaxer** Kneel close to the edge of a bed and lie face down with your abdomen and upper body resting on the bed's surface.
- **Stability Ball Back Relaxer** Lie face down on a stability ball with your feet and hands resting on the floor for balance.
- **Chair Forward Bend** Sit on a chair and let your back round by folding forwards. Let the arms dangle or – if the back feels stiff – rest your forearms on your knees.
- **Basic Lying Twist with Cushions** Perform a gentle lying twist (see Basic Lying Twist, page 49) and focus on relaxing the legs. Place cushions under the lower knee if your legs hover above the floor.
- **The Slouch Stretch** Sit with your legs stretched out in front. Relax your arms by your sides. Simply let your back round and let your head drop down. Notice where you feel the stretch: lower, mid or upper back. Just hold and breathe slowly through the nose.

SQUAT, DON'T BEND

It's instinctive to fold forwards from the lower back to pick up a dropped item or box from the floor, but doing this 'loads' the lower back as you straighten up. Providing your knees are healthy, try squatting instead. This places no pressure on your back and actually releases lower back tension. Squatting also lengthens and strengthens the calves and improves range of motion in the hip region.

Five-minute stretch sequences

String together some stretches into five-minute routines to keep the back mobile and supple.

Back sequence 1

1. STANDING TWIST

Stand with your feet hip-width apart. Bend your knees and relax your arms by your sides. Twist your upper body to the right and let the arms swing around. Return to the centre and twist to the left. Relax your arms and turn your head and torso as you rotate. *Repeat x 4.*

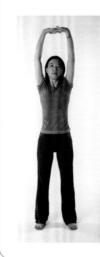

2. FULL BODY STRETCH

Stand with your feet hip-width apart. Sweep your arms up overhead and interlink your fingers. Press your palms towards the ceiling and remain here, drawing your shoulders downwards. *Hold for 10 seconds.*

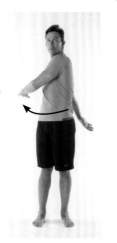

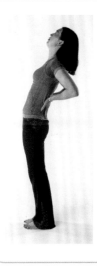

3. STANDING BACK BEND

Stand with your feet hip-width apart. Place your hands on your lower back, fingers pointing downwards. Stay looking forward or slightly down. Lean back. Push your hips forward. Draw your elbows together. *Hold for 10 seconds.*

4. STANDING UPPER BACK ROUNDER

Stand with your feet hip-width apart. Round your upper back and tuck your chin in. Sweep both arms forwards and interlock your fingers. *Hold for 10 seconds.*

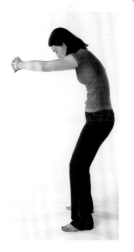

Back sequence 2

1. 90-DEGREE STRETCH

Stand with your feet hip-width apart. Tip your upper body forwards until you reach a 90-degree angle, or higher. Do not allow the back to curve. Draw the abdomen slightly inwards. Place your hands on your thighs just above your knees. *Hold for 20 seconds.*

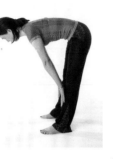

2. LOW LUNGE

Lower yourself down to all fours. Step your right foot up in between your hands and raise your upper body. Push your hips forward. Slowly lower into the lunge. *Hold for 20 seconds.*

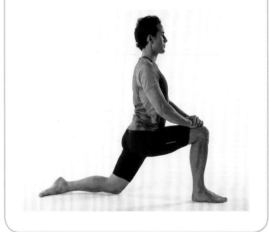

3. PELVIC TILT

Lie on your back with your legs bent and feet flat on the floor. Have your arms by your sides. Keep your hips on the floor throughout. First, tilt your pelvis up by pressing your lower back into the floor. Now tilt your pelvis back by lifting your belly button up to the ceiling. *Repeat x 4.*

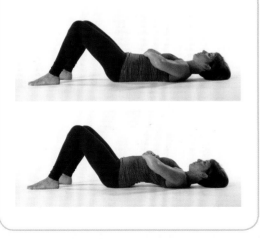

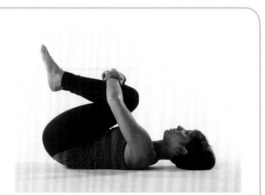

4. DOUBLE LEG HUG

Lie on your back and hug both legs into your abdomen. Rock a little from side to side across the lower back. *Hold for 10 seconds.*

Back sequence 3

1. CAT STRETCH

Start on all fours. As you inhale, lift your head and hips, allowing the mid back to dip.
As you exhale, tuck the chin and hips under allowing the back to round. *Repeat x 4.*

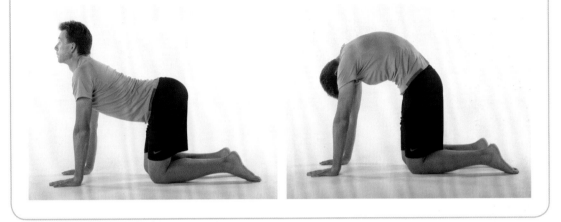

2. ALL FOURS MID-BACK TWIST

Start on all fours, but with your knees wide apart. Ensure your hands are directly
under your shoulders. Place your left hand on your left shoulder. Stay looking down.
As you inhale, point the left elbow up to the ceiling. As you exhale, point the left elbow
under the right armpit. Repeat on the other side. *Repeat x 4.*

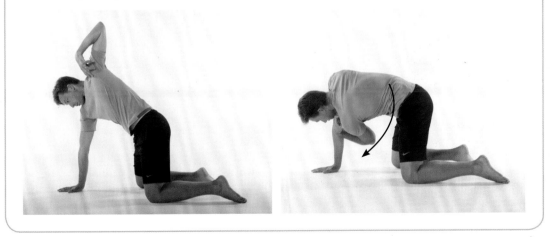

3. KNEELING BACK STRETCH WITH HOOKED THUMBS

On all fours, lower yourself down and sit on your heels. Reach your hands out in front of you and move them close together. Spread your fingers and press down. Hook your thumbs together. Draw your hips away in the opposite direction. *Hold for 20 seconds.*

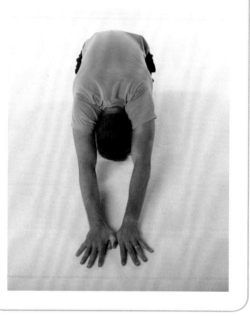

4. KNEELING SIDE STRETCH

Release your thumb hook in the Kneeling Back Stretch position. Walk your hands over to the right. Press the palms into the floor. *Hold for 30 seconds.* Walk your hands over to the left and press your palms into the floor. *Hold for 30 seconds.*

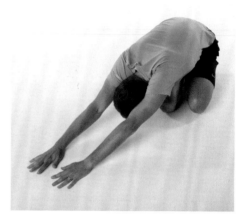

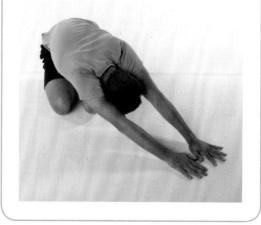

Back sequence 4

1. SPHINX

From all fours, lie down on your front positioning your elbows directly under your shoulders with the forearms parallel. Draw the shoulder blades slightly closer together. *Hold for 10 seconds.*

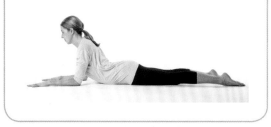

2. CHILD'S POSE

From all fours, lower yourself slowly down to sit back on your heels. Rest your forehead on the floor and relax your arms by your sides. If your forehead does not reach the floor, place some foam blocks or cushions under your forehead to raise the floor level. *Hold for 20 seconds.*

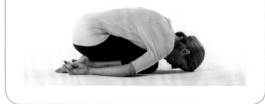

3. BASIC LYING TWIST

Lie on your back. Bend both legs and place your feet on the floor. Stretch your arms out at shoulder height, palms facing upwards. Lower both legs down to the floor on the right side and relax them. *Hold for 30 seconds.*

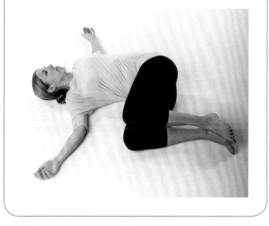

4. STRAP HAMSTRING STRETCH

Lie on your back and loop a strap, belt or tie around the sole of your right foot. Bend your left leg and place your foot on the floor. Straighten the right leg up towards the ceiling or keep it a little bent. *Hold for 30 seconds.* Repeat on the other side. *Hold for 30 seconds.*

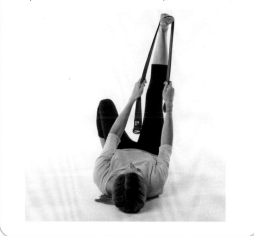

Stretches for the Hips and Buttocks

This chapter hones in on all the muscles of your hips and buttocks, from the hip flexors, found where the front of the thigh joins the pelvis, to the muscles at the sides of the hips and the larger buttocks or 'gluteus maximus'. Overly tight hip muscles can trigger problems both lower down in the knees and higher up in the lower back. Runners, cyclists and other endurance athletes are particularly prone to stiffness in this area as are people who spend long periods sitting at a desk or driving. Either target a particular area such as the hip flexors if you know that is a problem spot, or flick to the back of the section to follow a series of ready-made sequences to improve overall hip and glute flexibility.

THREE EVERYDAY WAYS TO GET SUPPLE HIPS

1 Sit on the sofa cross-legged or in Butterfly (see page 71).

2 Perform the Figure four stretch (see page 70) sitting at your desk.

3 Do a High Lunge (see page 67) pushing your hips forwards.

WARMING UP

Repeat each technique x 4

HIP CIRCLE
Place your hands on your hips and make large, smooth circles with your hips, keeping a slight bend in your knees.

HEEL TAP
Stand on your right leg. Lift your left leg up, bend it and turn your knee out. Tap your left heel with your right hand. Switch from leg to leg.

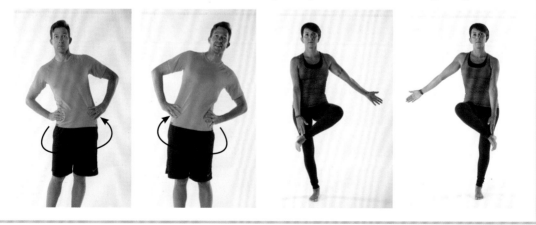

WARMING UP (CONT.)

Repeat each technique x 4

DYNAMIC SIDE BENDING

Stand with your feet hip-width apart. Sweep your left arm up and tip over to the right, trying not to lean forwards or backwards. Return to the centre. Sweep the right arm up and tip to the left.

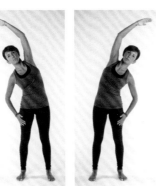

LUNGE

Place your hands on your hips. Take a large step forwards with your right leg and bend your knee to a 90-degree angle, ensuring the ankle is either directly under, or just behind your knee. Simultaneously drop your back knee down so that it hovers above the floor. Step back to standing. Switch from leg to leg.

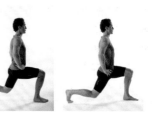

Front of hip stretches

Been told that your hip flexors need stretching? These muscles, which can be felt where the top of the thigh joins the pelvis, are often tight in runners, cyclists and other endurance athletes. But people who sit a lot can also benefit from hip flexor (or iliopsoas) stretching, especially as short, tight hip flexors can aggravate the lower back.

Lunging is the best way to stretch the front of the hips. Here are a few lunge variations:

LOW LUNGE

Lower yourself down to all fours. Step your right foot up in between your hands and raise your upper body. Push your hips forward. Slowly lower into the lunge.

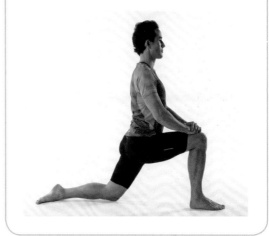

LOW LUNGE WITH CHEST STRETCH

Lower yourself down to all fours. Step your right foot up in between your hands and raise the upper body. Push your hips forwards and lower into the lunge. Take your hands behind your back and interlink your fingers. Draw your shoulders back and squeeze your shoulder blades closer.

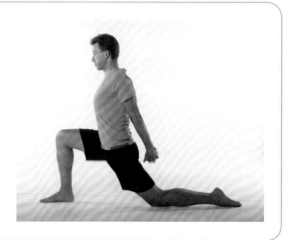

LOW LUNGE HIP POSITION

It is possible to almost miss out stretching the hip flexors in a low lunge if you fail to push your hips forward. In other words, don't do the stretch with your backside sticking out. Many people have trouble detecting the position of their pelvis so if you are unsure, reach around and slide a hand down your lower back. Rather than feeling the dip of your lower back or lumbar curve, you are aiming for a flatter lower back.

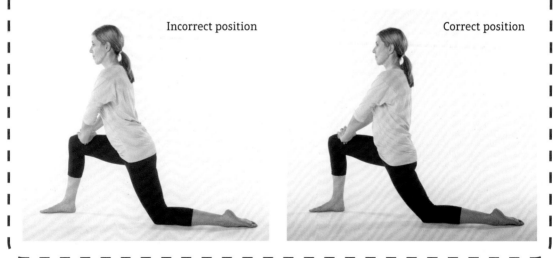

Incorrect position

Correct position

HIGH LUNGE

Stand with your feet hip-width apart and your hands on your hips. Take a large step back with your left foot and press your back heel down. Bend your left knee a little and push your hips forwards. Repeat on the other side.

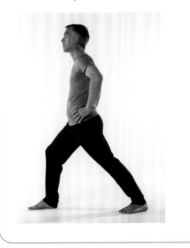

CHAIR HIGH LUNGE

Stand in front of a chair with your hands on your hips. Place your right foot on the chair and bend your right leg. Tuck the pelvis under or push your hips forward. Repeat on the other side.

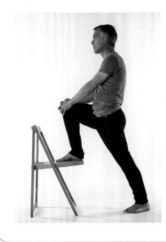

LIZARD

From all fours, step your right foot up to the outside of the right hand. Let your hips sink down. Either remain here with straight arms or slowly lower down onto the forearms. A block or book under each forearm will raise the floor level if this proves difficult. Repeat on the other side.

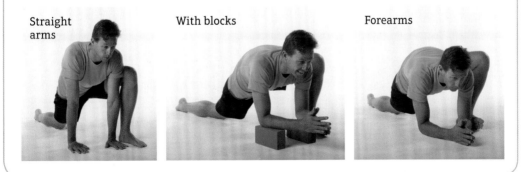

Straight arms

With blocks

Forearms

Outer hip and buttock stretches

When we talk about the 'glutes' we usually mean the biggest buttock muscle group or 'gluteus maximus', but there are smaller muscles on the sides of the hips which can benefit from stretching. Here are a few stretches to target the smaller gluteus medius that will also reach down the side of the upper thigh, encompassing the iliotibial band.

STANDING CROSSED-LEG STRETCH

Stand with your feet hip-width apart. Step your left foot over your right so the legs cross. Reach your left arm up and lean to the right.

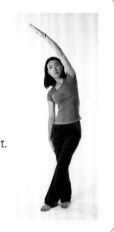

LOW LUNGE SIDE BEND

Start on all fours. Step your right foot up in between your hands and raise the upper body. Push your hips forwards. Lower into the lunge. Reach high with your left arm and lean the upper body to the right. Repeat on the other side.

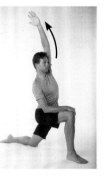

THE LEG KNOT

Sit with your legs out straight. Bend your right leg and step it over your left. Lean a little to the left, bend your left leg and slowly sit back down into the middle space. Both buttocks should be on the floor. If your body is tilted, unravel and practise the Seated Leg Hug (page 72) until hip flexibility improves. Place both hands just below the front knee and sit up straight. Repeat on the other side.

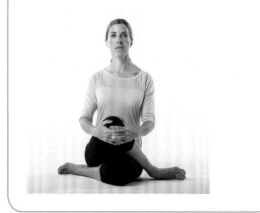

THE LEG KNOT TWIST

Perform The Leg Knot. Wrap your left arm around your right knee and place your right fingertips on the floor behind you. Sit tall. Rotate your upper body to the right in stages: lower back, mid back and head. Repeat on the other side.

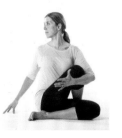

LYING LEG KNOT

Lie on your back with your legs bent. Cross your right leg over your left at thigh level and hug both legs in towards you. Hold just below your top knee or clasp both feet. Switch legs by crossing the left leg on top. Repeat on the other side.

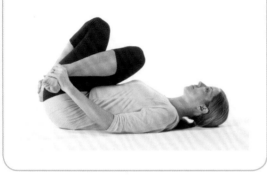

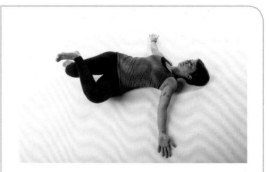

HOOKED LYING TWIST

Lie on your back with your legs bent and feet on the floor. Stretch your arms out at shoulder height, palms facing upwards. Lower both legs down to the floor on the left side. Slide your lower leg out and place your foot on top of the higher leg, just above your knee. Repeat on the other side.

LYING PIGEON

Lie on your back and draw your right leg in towards your chest. Hold onto your right knee with your left hand and draw your leg across your body. Repeat on the other side.

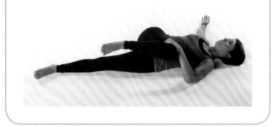

PIGEON

Start on all fours. Slide your right knee up behind your right wrist. Wiggle the right foot a little over to the left. Straighten the back leg. Lower yourself slowly either onto your forearms or stack one hand on top of the other and rest your forehead on your hands. Repeat on the other side.

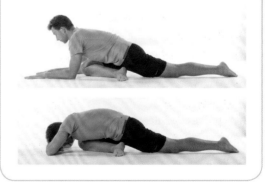

THE FIGURE FOUR STRETCH VARIATIONS

This effective stretch for the deep muscles of the buttocks can be done lying, standing or sitting. If sitting, experiment with the intensity of the stretch by leaning the upper body forwards or backwards. Figure Four Chair can be done anywhere: at the office or on the daily train commute, without anyone knowing you are undertaking hip flexibility training!

1. FIGURE FOUR

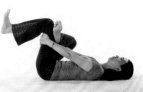

Lie on your back with your legs bent. Lift your right foot of the floor and turn your knee out. Rest your right ankle on top of your left thigh. Stay here or draw both legs in towards you. Hold behind the front thigh or clasp the front shin. Repeat on the other side. *Hold for 30 seconds.*

2. FIGURE FOUR SITTING

Sit on the floor with your legs bent. Lift your right foot off the floor and turn your knee out. Rest your right ankle on top of your left thigh. Stay here or lift the feet off the floor and draw both legs in towards you. Hold behind the front thigh or clasp the front shin. If your

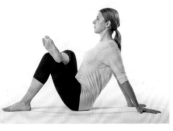

head tilts back, elevate it on blocks or cushions. Repeat on the other side.

To move deeper into the Figure Four sitting stretch try drawing the legs in closer, holding for a 5-10 seconds, then repeating twice more.

3. FIGURE FOUR STANDING

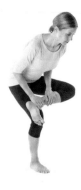

You may want to do this stretch close to a chair or wall for support. Stand with your feet hip-width apart. Bend both legs, lift your left leg off the floor, turn your knee out and lay your left ankle on top of your right thigh. To go deeper, squat lower. Repeat on the other side.

4. FIGURE FOUR CHAIR

Sit on a chair with a straight back and both feet on the floor. Lift your left foot off the floor and turn your knee out.

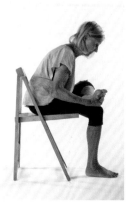

Rest your left ankle on top of your right thigh. Keeping the back straight, lean the upper body forwards a little. Lean further forwards to increase the intensity of the stretch. Repeat on the other side.

Groin stretches

These stretches target the muscles of the inner thighs and groin in a variety of sitting and lying positions. This section ends with the classic cross-legged position and a step-by-step guide to achieving it if you struggle with hip flexibility.

DIAMOND

Sit with a straight back, perching on the edge of a cushion if this makes it more comfortable. Bring the soles of your feet together but move them further away until the legs form a diamond shape. Keeping your back straight, lean your upper body forwards.

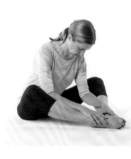

BUTTERFLY

Sit down and place the soles of your feet together. Either clasp your hands around the feet or hold onto your ankles and sit taller. To move deeper into the stretch, keep your back straight and lean your upper body forwards.

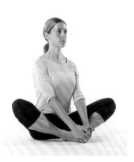

DON'T BOUNCE THE BUTTERFLY

A dynamic version of Butterfly exists whereby the legs are bounced (or wings flapped) rapidly. Such a sharp, quick movement is likely to trigger a contract response in the muscles of the groin and inner thighs – the exact opposite to the slow muscular release we want. Instead, hold the stretch steady, breathe deeply through the nose and wait for the inner thigh muscles to relax. Over time, the legs will drop closer to the floor.

TORTOISE

Sit with your legs in a diamond shape and the soles of your feet together. Let your upper body drop forwards so your back rounds and your head hangs down. Rest your forearms on your legs or hold onto your feet.

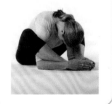

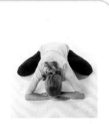

FROG

Come to all fours. Position your knees wide and bring your toes to touch. Lower back to sit on your heels. Stack one hand one top of the other and rest your forehand on your hands.

HOW TO SIT CROSS-LEGGED

If you haven't sat on the floor since the age of seven or eight at school, your hips are unlikely to drop easily into a cross-legged position. Your knees may stick up causing you to tip back. The back is then forced to keep your body upright, resulting in an aching lower back. Essentially the cross-legged position will only really be comfortable when you can get your knees lower. Then the pelvis can tilt forwards and the back can lengthen. The trick is to begin by elevating the hips or pelvis on either a yoga block or two, or a few cushions. If your knees are still off the floor, place cushions under them too. Sitting against a wall will also help support the back. Why bother sitting cross-legged? With your knees resting on the floor, it is a very balanced way to sit with a straight back and will create a stable tripod-shaped base that allows you to breathe or meditate in comfort. It also stretches the muscles around your groin and buttocks, and strengthens the back. But it requires a little dedication. If sitting cross-legged proves impossible don't worry; substitute a more accessible groin stretch such as Butterfly (page 71) or Diamond (page 71).

Here is a five-step plan to sitting cross-legged:

1. SEATED LEG HUG

Sit with your legs out straight. Bend your right leg and step it over your left. Wrap both arms around your leg and hug it into your body. Sit up straight. Repeat on the other side.

2. LEG CRADLE

Sit on the floor with both legs straight. Cradle one leg by placing one hand on your foot and one just below your knee. Sit up straight. Either hold the leg still or rock it slowly from side to side.

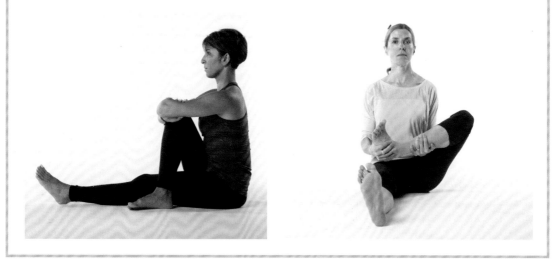

HOW TO SIT CROSS-LEGGED (CONT.)

3. BUTTERFLY

Sit with a straight back, perching on the edge of a cushion or two if this makes it more comfortable. Bring the soles of your feet together. Either clasp your hands around the feet or hold onto your ankles and sit taller. To move deeper into the stretch, keep your back straight and lean the upper body forwards.

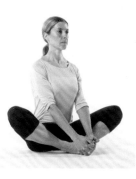

4. DIAMOND

Sit with a straight back, perching on the edge of a cushion or two if this makes it more comfortable. Bring the soles of your feet together but move them further away until the legs form a diamond shape. Keeping your back straight, lean the upper body forwards.

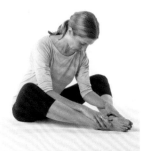

5. SITTING CROSS-LEGGED

Sit with a straight back, cross the right leg in front of the left. Remember to alternate which foot you position in front if you practise sitting cross-legged regularly.

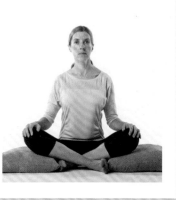

Is One Hip Stiffer than the Other?

If the answer is 'yes', then you are not alone. It is relatively common to have one stiffer hip. This will be obvious when you come to perform the Figure Four stretch (see page 70) as firstly it may be a struggle simply to get into the start position on the tighter side, and secondly, the top knee may be closer to your body so the whole stretch feels more cramped. Perform the stretch regularly and hold a little longer on the stiffer side.

Five-minute stretch sequences

String together some stretches into five-minute routines for improved flexibility in the hips and buttocks region.

Hips and buttocks sequence 1

1. HIP CIRCLE

Stand with your feet hip-width apart. Place your hands on your hips and make large, smooth circles with your hips keeping a slight bend in your knees. *Repeat x 4.*

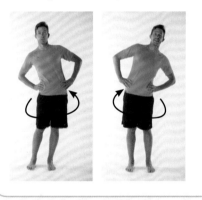

2. STANDING CROSSED-LEG STRETCH

Stand with your feet hip-width apart. Step your left foot over your right so the legs cross and lean to the left. To deepen this stretch, reach your left arm over by your ear. *Hold for 10 seconds.* Repeat on the other side. *Hold for 10 seconds.*

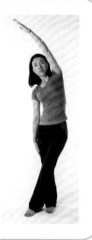

3. CHAIR HIGH LUNGE

Stand in front of a chair with your hands on your hips. Place your right foot on the chair and bend your right leg a little. Push your hips forwards. *Hold for 20 seconds.* Repeat on the other side. *Hold for 20 seconds.*

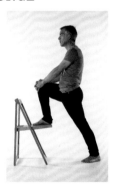

4. FIGURE FOUR CHAIR

Sit on a chair with a straight back and both feet on the floor. Lift your left foot off the floor and turn your knee out. Rest your left ankle on top of your right thigh. Keeping the back straight, lean the upper body forwards a little. Lean further forwards to increase the intensity of the stretch. *Hold for 20 seconds.* Repeat on the other side. *Hold for 20 seconds.*

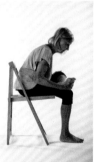

Hips and buttocks sequence 2

1. LOW LUNGE

Lower yourself down to all fours. Step your right foot up in between your hands and raise your upper body. Push your hips forward. Slowly lower into the lunge. *Hold for 20 seconds.* Repeat on the other side. *Hold for 20 seconds.*

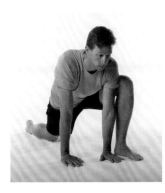

2. LOW LUNGE WITH SIDE BEND

From the Low Lunge, reach high with your left arm and lean the upper body over to the right. *Hold for 20 seconds.* Repeat on the other side. *Hold for 20 seconds.*

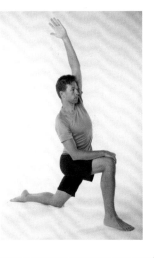

3. LIZARD

From all fours, step your left foot up to the outside of the left hand. Let your hips sink down. Either remain with straight arms or slowly lower down onto the forearms. A block or book under each forearm will raise the floor level if this proves difficult. *Hold for 30 seconds.* Repeat on the other side. *Hold for 30 seconds.*

4. PIGEON

From the Lizard, wriggle your right foot a little over to the left. Straighten your back leg. Lower yourself slowly either onto your forearms or stack one hand on top of the other and rest your forehead on your hands. *Hold for 30 seconds.* Repeat on the other side. *Hold for 30 seconds.*

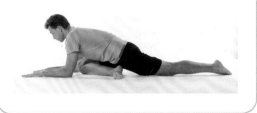

Hips and buttocks sequence 3

1. SEATED LEG HUG

Sit with your legs out straight. Bend your right leg and step it over your left. Wrap both arms around your leg and hug it into your body. Sit up straight. *Hold for 20 seconds.* Repeat on the other side. *Hold for 20 seconds.*

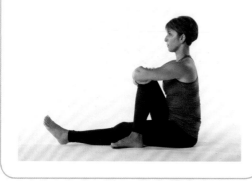

2. LEG CRADLING STRETCH

Sit with your legs out straight. Bend your left leg and draw it closer to your body. Cradle the leg by placing one hand on your foot and one just below your knee. Sit up straight. Either hold the leg still or rock it slowly from side to side. *Hold for 10 seconds.* Repeat on the other side. *Hold for 10 seconds.*

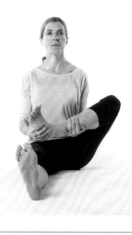

3. BUTTERFLY

Sit with a straight back, perching on the edge of a cushion or two if this makes it more comfortable. Bring the soles of your feet together. Either clasp your hands around the feet or hold onto your ankles and sit taller. *Hold for 20 seconds.*

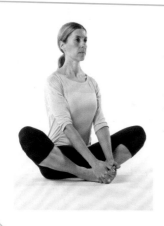

4. TORTOISE

Move your legs further away so they form a diamond shape. Let your upper body drop forwards so your back rounds and your head hangs down. Rest your forearms on your legs or hold onto your feet. *Hold for 20 seconds.*

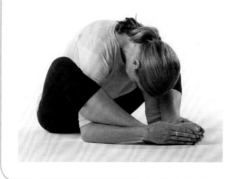

Hips and buttocks sequence 4

1. SINGLE LEG HUG

Lie on your back and draw your right leg in towards your chest. Keep your left leg straight and press the back of the left knee into the floor. *Hold for 20 seconds.* Repeat on the other side. *Hold for 20 seconds.*

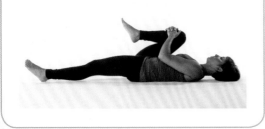

2. LYING PIGEON

Lie on your back and draw your right leg into your abdomen. Hold onto your right knee with your left hand and draw your leg across your body. *Hold for 30 seconds.* Repeat on the other side. *Hold for 30 seconds.*

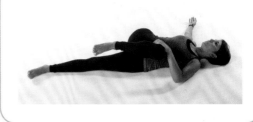

3. FIGURE FOUR

Lie on your back with your legs bent. Lift your right foot off the floor and turn your knee out. Rest your right ankle on top of your left thigh. Stay here or lift the feet off the floor and draw both legs in towards you. Hold behind the front thigh or clasp the front shin. If your head tilts back elevate it on blocks or cushions. *Hold for 30 seconds.* Repeat on the other side. *Hold for 30 seconds.*

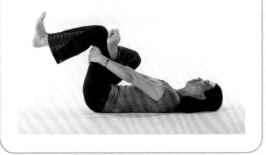

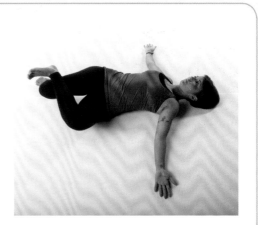

4. HOOKED LYING TWIST

Lie with your legs bent and feet on the floor. Stretch your arms out shoulder-height, palms facing upwards. Lower both legs down to the floor on the left side. Slide your lower leg out and place your foot on top of the higher leg, just above your knee. *Hold for 30 seconds.*

Stretches for the Upper Legs

This chapter targets the following leg muscles: the hamstrings (at the back of the thigh), the quadriceps (at the front of the thigh), the adductors (inner thigh), the abductors (outer thigh), and the muscles and tendons which run down the outside of the upper leg from the hip to the knee, such as the iliotibial band. Handpick a series of stretches to suit you, from chair-based to kneeling for a particular muscle group, or try a ready-made sequence for the overall upper leg region from the end of this chapter.

WARMING UP

Repeat each technique x 4

LEG SWING

Stand on your left leg and slowly swing your right leg back and forth. Let your arms swing freely 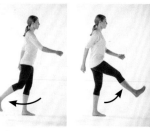 in opposition to mimic walking or running or place your hand on a surface for balance. Repeat on the other side.

SIDE LEG SWING

Stand on your left leg and slowly swing your right leg across your body back and 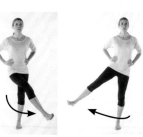 forth. Rest your left hand on a wall for support if required. Repeat on the other side.

BACK KICKS

Stand on your right leg. Bend your left leg as if lifting your heel to your buttocks. Switch from leg to leg.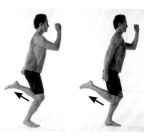

SUMO SQUAT

Place your hands on your thighs. Step your feet wide with your toes slightly turned outwards. Bend both legs and lower into a squat, checking that your knees are aligned with your second toes and your toes are just visible in the squat. Rise back up to standing.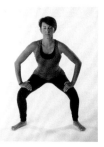

The Hamstrings

Many people complain about having tight hamstrings and are frustrated by their inability to touch their toes. My response to this is that toe touching should not always be the main goal when lengthening these muscles at the back of the thigh. Firstly, it is not the best hamstring flexibility test and, secondly, pushing your hands down to your feet may strain your lower back. The good news is that there are 101 ways to stretch the hamstrings that would suit everyone from the less flexible to the bendiest yogi. Before you start, gauge your own levels of hamstring flexibility by trying the Waiter's Bow test (see page 80). If you feel you belong in the 'tight hamstring' group, read Six Rules for Stretching Tight Hamstrings below before you get started.

SIX RULES FOR STRETCHING TIGHT HAMSTRINGS

1 Bend Your Knees If performing a sitting or standing hamstring stretch, bending your knees a little will relieve the strain both on the hamstrings and lower back.

2 Sit on a Cushion Perching right on the edge on a cushion or foam yoga block will tip the pelvis forward which relieves the pull on the hamstrings and is more comfortable for the lower back.

3 Watch Your Back If you have a weak or injured lower back, keep your back straight when hamstring stretching. Lie on your back and loop a strap around your foot or try the Waiter's Bow (see page 80). There are no prizes for pushing your nose to your knees.

4 Use a Strap Obtain a cotton yoga strap, dressing gown belt or old tie for seated or lying hamstring stretches to reduce strain and ensure proper alignment.

5 Be Patient Hold the stretch for 20-30 seconds. Use this time to tune into your breathing and relax.

6 Don't Strain Never push into the stretch or move beyond your natural limit as the muscles will contract in response and you may even damage your hamstrings. Find the 'edge' of the stretch and wait until there is a little space to move deeper.

TEST YOUR HAMSTRING FLEXIBILITY: THE WAITER'S BOW

The traditional way of assessing hamstring flexibility is the Sit and Reach test: sitting with the legs outstretched and reaching forwards to grab your toes. However, this only partially assesses how bendy your lower back is and may even strain the lower back region. The Waiter's Bow technique removes this curving of the back to focus purely on the hamstrings. Simply stand tall with the feet hip-width apart. Place your right hand on your lower back and feel the dip or curve. Maintain that curve throughout the stretch. Now place your left palm on your abdomen and begin to tip forwards from the hips while keeping the back straight. A bend of 90 degrees or beyond is considered flexible, but perform regularly, three times a week or more, holding for 30 seconds and repeating three times, to see gradual improvements. Remember to exit the stretch by bending your knees and pulling in the stomach before you rise up to a standing position.

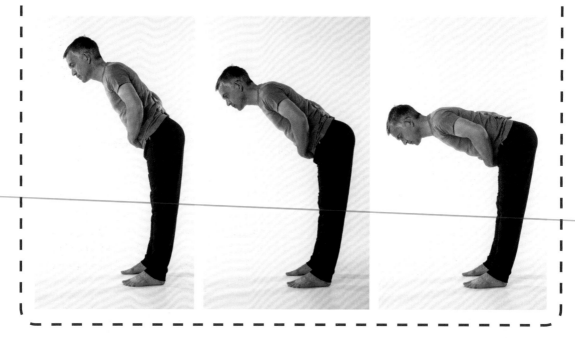

Standing hamstring stretches

LEAN FORWARD STRETCH

From a standing position, take a small step back with your left leg. Bend your left leg and tip your upper body forwards, placing both hands on your right thigh. Press the sole of the left foot into the floor. Repeat on the other side.

LEG UP CHAIR STRETCH

Put your right foot on the seat of a chair (or a lower surface, such as a step). Stand tall with your hands on your hips. Tip your upper body forwards until you feel the hamstrings stretching. Repeat on the other side.

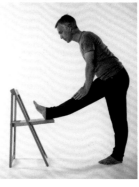

90-DEGREE STRETCH

Stand with your feet hip-width apart. Tip your upper body forwards until you reach a 90-degree angle, or higher. Do not allow the back to curve. Draw the abdomen slightly inwards. Place your hand on your thighs just above your knees.

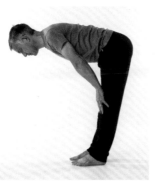

90-DEGREE CHAIR STRETCH

Stand behind a chair and place your hands on the top of the chair back, shoulder-width apart. Walk backwards until you fold into a 90-degree position. Move your head in line with the spine. To exit, walk forwards, bend your knees, draw the abdomen in and rise up to standing. This stretch can also be done at a kitchen counter.

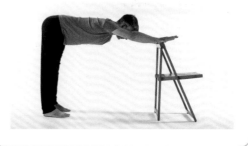

FULL FORWARD BEND

Stand with the feet hip-width apart and a slight bend in your knees. Fold forward and place either your fingertips or palms on the floor either side of your feet. Exit carefully by bending your knees deeper, pulling in your abdomen and rising up to standing with a straight back.

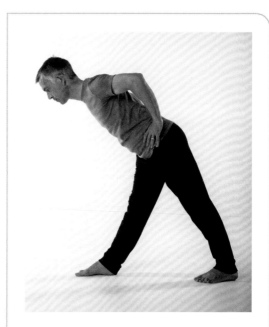

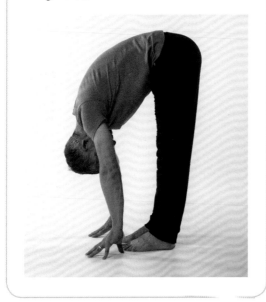

HALF PYRAMID STRETCH

Stand with your feet hip-width apart and place your hands on your hips. Take a step back with your left foot. Tip your upper body forwards until you reach a 45-degree angle or lower. You may need to bend the front knee slightly. Repeat on the other side.

FULL PYRAMID STRETCH

Stand with your feet hip-width apart. Take a step back with your left foot. Tip your upper body forwards and place your palms or fingertips on the floor, either side of the front foot. Repeat on the other side.

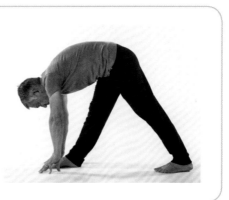

Seated hamstring stretches

SEATED HAMSTRING STRAP STRETCH

Sit with your legs straight. Perch on the edge of a cushion or bend your knees slightly if this is difficult. Loop a strap, tie or dressing gown belt around your feet. Remain sitting upright or tilt the upper body forwards without rounding the back.

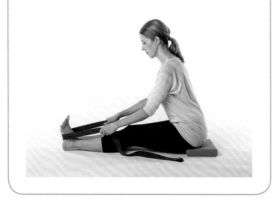

SEATED HAMSTRING AND HIP STRAP STRETCH

Sit with your legs straight. Bend your left leg and place the sole of your left foot into your inner right thigh. Sit up straight (perch on the edge of a cushion or bend your knees slightly if this is difficult). Loop a strap around your right foot. Remain sitting upright or tilt the upper body forwards without rounding the back. Repeat on the other side.

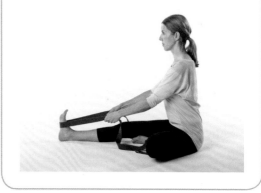

Stretch the Hamstrings, Not the Back

Lower back pain is often accompanied by tight hamstrings. However, many folding forwards positions can aggravate back problems. Keep the natural curve in the lower back as you stretch. Sitting on a cushion will tip the pelvis forwards and ease the pressure on the lower back in seated positions. Or try one of the following stretches:

- Lean Forward Stretch (page 81)

- 90-Degree Stretch (page 81)

- Lying Hamstring Strap Stretch (page 84)

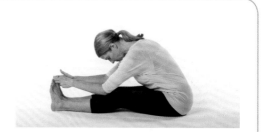

ADVANCED SEATED HAMSTRING STRETCH

Sit up straight. Fold forward, aiming to bring your chest towards your knees rather than pushing the nose to your knees. If comfortable, hold onto your toes or feet.

Lying hamstring stretches

SINGLE LEG HUG

Lie on your back and draw your right leg in towards your chest. Keep your left leg straight and press the back of your left knee into the floor. Repeat on the other side.

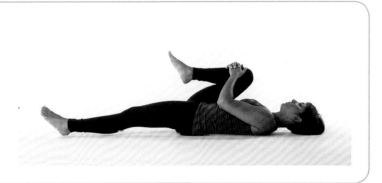

LYING HAMSTRING STRAP STRETCH

Lie on your back and loop a strap, belt or tie around the sole of your right foot. Bend your left leg and place your foot on the floor, especially if your hamstrings are tight. Straighten your right leg or bend it a little. Repeat on the other side.

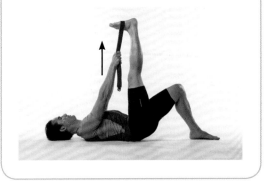

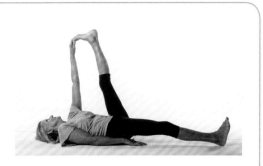

ADVANCED LYING HAMSTRING STRETCH

Lie on your back. Lift your left leg up towards the ceiling. Straighten your right leg and rest it on the floor. Hold behind your thigh and draw your leg closer towards you. You may be able to walk your hands higher up to your foot or grasp your toes with your left hand. Repeat on the other side.

The Inner Thighs

The inner thighs or adductors can become stiff or tight due to inactivity or overuse potentially causing knock-on problems with the hips and lower back. Sportspeople such as footballers who perform a lot of lateral (side to side) movement using these muscles are also susceptible to groin strain and should include one or two adductor stretches in every post-match stretching session to avoid injury.

CHAIR INNER THIGH STRETCH

Stand next to a chair with the seat facing toward you. Lift your right leg up and place your right foot on the seat. Place your hand on your hips. Keep your toes facing forward.

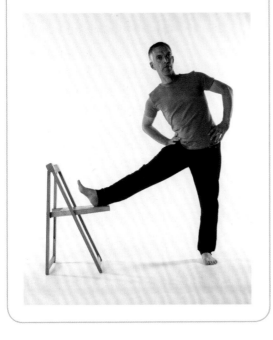

WIDE-LEGGED FORWARD BEND

From a standing position, step your feet wide and turn your toes slightly inwards. Place your hands on your hips and tip your upper body forwards, stopping when your back begins to round. Remain here, or place your hands on the floor.

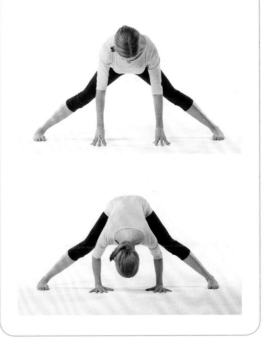

WIDE-LEGGED SEATED STRETCH

Sit tall with your legs stretched out wide and toes pointing upward. Keeping a straight spine, begin to walk your hands forwards until you feel your back and inner thigh muscles stretching.

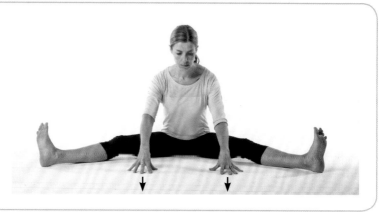

SIDE LUNGE

Step your feet wide apart with your toes slightly turned out. Bend your right knee and lower over to the right but ensure that your right knee stays behind your right foot (you can still see your toes). Pause here. Rise up and repeat on the other side.

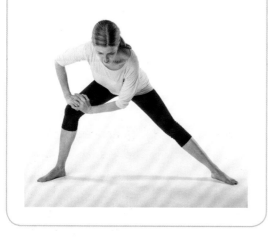

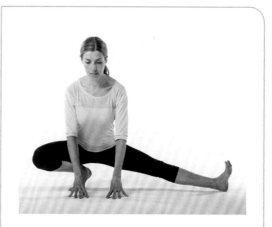

COSSACK STRETCH

Step your feet wide apart with your toes slightly turned out. Bend your right leg and slowly lower yourself all the way to the floor until your buttocks reach your right heel. Now turn your left toes upwards and try to lower the heel you are kneeling on. Rest your fingertips on the floor. Repeat on the other side.

For more inner thigh stretches, turn to The Hips section (page 64).

The Quadriceps

While there are a huge range of hamstring stretches, there are less ways to access the four quadriceps or 'quads' located at the front of the thigh, but here is a variety that I hope will suit everyone, whatever their range of motion. If extreme flexion of your knee, such as kneeling, is uncomfortable, please stick to stretches which place less pressure on your knee joint such as Side Lying Quad Stretch, and hook a strap, belt or tie around the foot if it proves hard to grasp.

Standing quad stretches

STANDING QUAD STRETCH

Stand tall with your feet hip-width apart. Slowly bend your right leg and reach around to hold the foot with your right hand. Your knee should be pointing downward. Hold onto a chair for balance if required. Push your hips forward. Repeat on the other side.

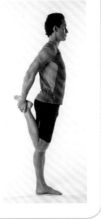

ANCHORED QUAD STRETCH

Stand with your back to a chair. Lift your left leg up behind you and hook your toes onto the the back of the chair (if the chair back is too high, try a lower surface such as a table). Bend your right leg a little and push your hips forward. Repeat on the other side.

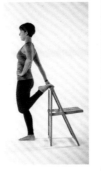

DYNAMIC QUAD STRETCH

Stand tall with your feet hip-width apart. Slowly bend your right leg and reach around to hold your foot with your right hand. Push your hips forward. Bend your standing leg and draw your right leg back further. Now start to move your leg by alternately pointing your knee forward and drawing your knee back. Repeat on the other side. *Repeat x 4* .

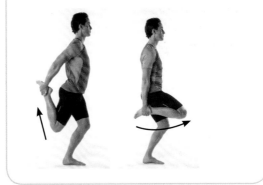

Moving Deeper in a Quad Stretch

If you feel like you have the space to go deeper into your thigh stretch, try the Standing Quad Stretch, Lying Quad Stretch (page 89), or All Fours Quad Stretch (page 88). First, push the front of your foot into your hand. Now draw your heel closer to your buttocks. You can repeat these steps a few times to bring your heel closer.

Floor-based quad stretches

ALL FOURS QUAD STRETCH

Start on all fours with your fingers spread wide. Lean to the right, placing your left hand on your left knee and sliding your hand down to your foot. Now gently draw the leg back. Repeat on the other side.

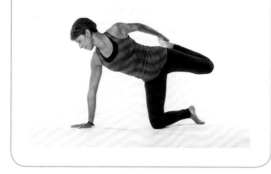

LOW LUNGE

Start on all fours. Step your right foot up in between your hands and raise your upper body. Push your hips forward. Slowly lower into the lunge. Repeat on the other side.

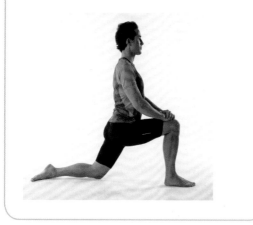

LOW LUNGE WITH QUAD STRETCH

If you are comfortable bearing weight on your back knee, try performing a low lunge combined with a quad stretch. Please note: you will need to be supple enough to sink the hips low enough so that most of the weight on the back knee is just above the joint, rather than on the kneecap itself. Do pad the back knee with a cushion or block.

Perform the low lunge with your right foot in front. Now lean a little to the right, and bend your left leg. Reach around to hold the left foot. Shift your weight back to the centre and lift your upper body. Either hold still or do the following steps:

- Press the front of your foot into your hand.
- Draw your heel closer to your body.

If you feel balanced, end by reaching around to the foot with the left hand too, drawing back your shoulders and lifting your chest. Then repeat on the other side.

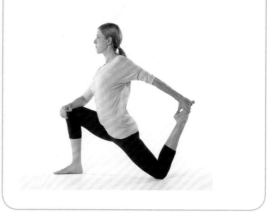

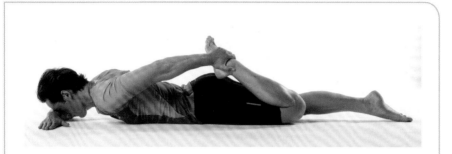

LYING QUAD STRETCH

Lower down onto your front. Bend your left leg and reach around for your foot. Press your hips into the floor to avoid arching the back and draw the leg closer to your buttocks. If you cannot reach the foot, loop a strap or tie around it. Repeat on the other side.

SIDE LYING QUAD STRETCH

Lie on your right side with your right leg a little bent under you for balance. Bend your left leg and reach for the foot. Push your hips forward. If you can't reach your foot, loop a strap or tie around it. Repeat on the other side.

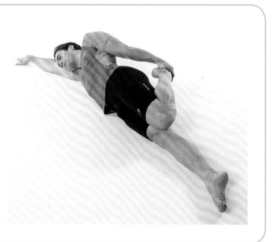

The kneeling series

1. KNEELING

Come to a kneeling position by sitting back onto your heels. This can be made more comfortable if you place three or four cushions between your buttocks and heels to raise your hips off the floor.

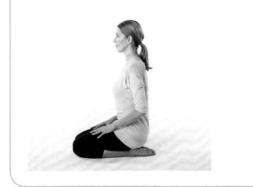

2. KNEELING WITH LIFT

In a kneeling position, place your hands behind you, press them into the floor and raise the hips up as high as you can. Either hold for 10-20 seconds and lower or work dynamically by breathing in to lift and breathing out to lower and repeating six times.

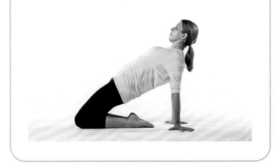

WARNING: KNEELING AND KNEE PAIN

Simply kneeling is a gentle way of lengthening the quadriceps, but if you have had a knee injury, surgery or are simply stiff around the joint, sitting in this position of 'full flexion' will be impossible or uncomfortable. The more advanced kneeling variations, which combine kneeling with lying back on the forearms, are best avoided if you have knee issues as they place undue pressure on the joint and surrounding ligaments. Sitting on a few cushions will widen the angle of your knees, making it more accessible. Or opt instead for the Low Lunge, maybe padding the back knee with a cushion. Other alternatives are the lower impact stretches, Standing Quad Stretch or Side Lying Quad Stretch.

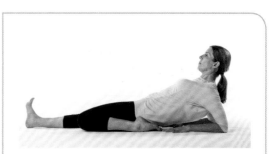

3. KNEELING LEAN BACK

Start in a kneeling position. Release your right leg and flex your right foot. Slowly and carefully lie back to rest either on your forearms or lower all the way to the floor and rest on your back.

Five-minute stretch sequences

String together some stretches into five-minute routines for improved flexibility in the upper leg region.

Upper leg sequence 1

1. LEG SWING

Stand on your right leg and slowly swing your left leg back and forth. Let your arms swing freely in opposition to mimic walking or running or place your hand on a surface for balance. *Repeat x 4*. Switch legs.

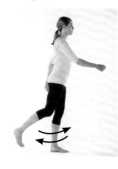

2. 90-DEGREE STRETCH

Stand with your feet hip-width apart. Tip your upper body forwards until you reach a 90-degree angle, or higher. Do not allow your back to curve. Draw your abdomen slightly inwards. Place your hand on your thighs just above your knees. *Hold for 20 seconds.*

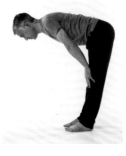

3. LOW LUNGE

Start on all fours. Step your right foot up in between your hands and raise your upper body. Push your hips forward. Slowly sink the hips lower into the lunge. *Hold for 20 seconds.*

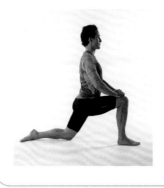

4. SEATED HAMSTRING AND HIP STRAP STRETCH

Bend your left leg and place the sole of your left foot into your inner right thigh. Sit up straight or perch on the edge of a cushion or bend your knees slightly if this is difficult. Loop a strap around your right foot. Remain sitting upright or tilt your upper body forwards without rounding your back. *Hold for 30 seconds.*

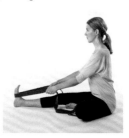

Upper leg sequence 2

1. BACK KICKS

Stand on your left leg. Bend your right leg as if lifting your heel to your buttocks. Switch from leg to leg. *Repeat x 8.*

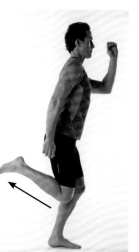

2. STANDING QUAD STRETCH

Stand tall with your feet hip-width apart. Slowly bend your right leg and reach around to hold your foot with your right hand. Your knee should be pointing downward. Reach your left arm out to the side or hold onto a chair for balance. Push your hips forward. *Hold for 20 seconds.*

3. HALF PYRAMID STRETCH

Stand with your feet hip-width apart and place your hands on your hips. Take a step back with your left foot. Tip your upper body forwards until you reach a 45-degree angle or higher. You may need to bend the front knee slightly. Repeat on the other side. *Hold for 30 seconds.*

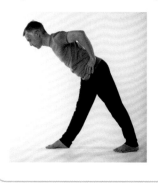

4. WIDE-LEGGED FORWARD BEND

From a standing position, step the feet wide and turn your toes slightly inwards. Place your hands on your hips and tip your upper body forwards, stopping when your back begins to round. Remain here, or place your hands on the floor. *Hold for 30 seconds.*

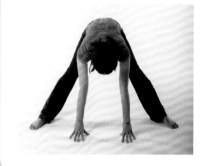

Upper leg sequence 3

1. SUMO SQUATS

Place your hands on your hips. Step your feet wide with your toes slightly turned outwards. Bend both legs and lower into a squat checking that your knees are aligned with your toes and your toes are just visible in the squat. Rise back up to a standing position. *Repeat x 4.*

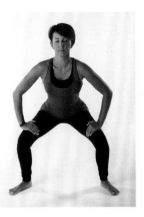

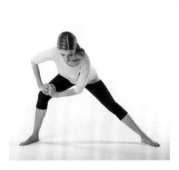

2. SIDE LUNGES

Step your feet wide apart with your toes slightly turned out. Bend your right knee and lower over to the right but ensure that your right knee stays behind your right foot and you can still see your toes. Pause here. Rise up and repeat on the other side. *Repeat x 4.*

3. LYING QUAD STRETCH

Lie down onto your front. Bend your left leg and reach around for your foot. Press your pelvis into the floor to avoid arching your back and draw your leg closer to your buttocks. Note: if you cannot reach the foot, loop a strap or tie around it. *Hold for 30 seconds.*

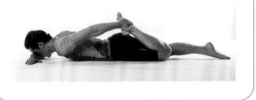

4. LYING HAMSTRING STRAP STRETCH

Lie on your back and loop a strap, belt or tie around the sole of your right foot. Bend the left leg and place the foot on the floor, especially if your hamstrings are tight. Straighten your right leg or bend it a little. Repeat on the other side. *Hold for 30-60 seconds.*

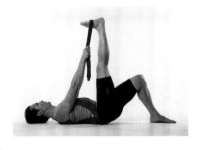

Upper leg sequence 4

1. 90-DEGREE CHAIR STRETCH

Stand behind a chair and place your hands on the top of the chair back, shoulder-width apart. Walk backwards until you fold into a 90-degree position. Move your head in line with your spine. Tuck your pelvis slightly under to flatten your lower back. To exit, walk forwards, bend your knees, draw your abdomen in and rise up to standing. This stretch can also be done at a kitchen counter. *Hold for 30 seconds.*

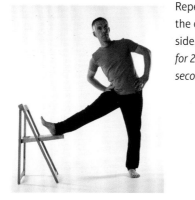

2. LEG UP CHAIR STRETCH

Put your right foot on the seat of a chair (or a lower surface, such as a step). Stand tall with your hands on your hips. Tip your upper body forwards until you feel your hamstrings stretching. Repeat on the other side. *Hold for 20 seconds.*

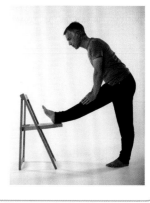

3. CHAIR INNER THIGH STRETCH

Stand next to a chair with the seat facing toward you. Lift your right leg up and place your right foot on the seat. Place your hands on your hips. Keep your toes facing forward. Repeat on the other side. *Hold for 20 seconds.*

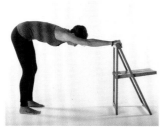

4. ANCHORED QUAD STRETCH

Stand with your back to a chair. Lift your left leg up behind you and hook your toes onto the top of the back of the chair. If the chair back is too high, try a lower surface such as a table. Bend your right leg a little and push your hips forward. Repeat on the other side. *Hold for 20 seconds.*

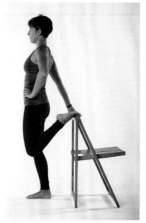

Stretches for The Lower Legs and Feet

The lower legs and feet carry the weight of the whole body when standing or walking. This can result in soreness around the soles of the feet, ankles, calves or shins. Sitting down and gently stretching the feet can greatly relieve this discomfort. For athletes, especially runners, it is vital to keep the lower legs strong and supple to absorb the shock of running and avoid suffering a twisted ankle or repetitive strain injury such as plantar fasciitis.

WARMING UP

Repeat each sequence x 4

ANKLE ROLL

Place your hands on your hips. Stand on your left leg and lift your right foot off the floor. Rotate your foot slowly. Switch feet.

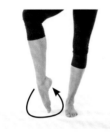

HEEL AND TOE ROCKING

Rock your weight back into the heels and lift your toes off the floor. Rock your weight forwards onto the balls of your feet and lift your heels off the floor.

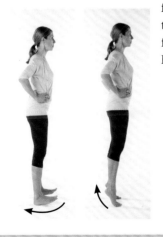

WALKING DOG

Start on all fours. Spread your fingers wide. Lift your hips up to make a triangle shape with your body. Bend one leg and push the other heel towards the floor. Continue, switching from side to side or pause for 10 seconds on each leg.

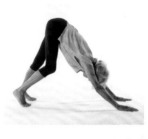

POINT AND FLEX

Sit with your legs stretched out in front of you and your feet hip-width apart. Alternately point your toes and flex your feet by drawing your toes back and pushing your heels forward.

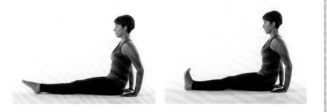

The Calves

The calves at the back of the lower leg feature two main muscles: the larger gastrocnemius, which bulges visibly in those with well-defined calves, and the smaller, flatter muscle soleus, which lies underneath. Both connect with the Achilles tendon, which extends down to the heel. Calf stretching is vital for people who favour sports with repetitive movements, such as runners or hikers, or athletes doing sudden explosive movements like jumping or lunging (basketball or tennis).

Standing calf stretches

STANDING TOES UP STRETCH

Take a step back with your left leg. Bend your left leg and tip your upper body forwards. Lift your right toes up to roll your foot on the heel.

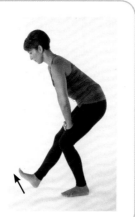

HIGH LUNGE

Stand with your feet hip-width apart and your hands on your hips. Take a large step back with your left foot and press your back heel down. Bend your right knee a little and push your hips forwards. Repeat on the other side.

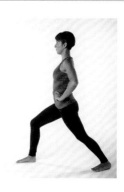

STEP OR BLOCK STRETCH

Stand on the edge of the stairs or a couple of foam yoga blocks or books. Keep your left leg straight and drop the left heel off the edge of the platform. Switch from side to side.

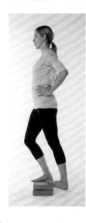

DOUBLE STEP OR BLOCK STRETCH

Stand on the edge of the stairs or a couple of foam yoga blocks or books. Keep both legs straight and drop both heels off the edge of the platform. Lean a little forward.

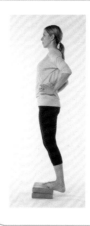

The dog stretches

WALKING DOG

Start on all fours. Spread your fingers wide. Lift your hips up to make a triangle shape with your body. Bend one leg and push the other heel towards the floor. Continue, switching from side to side or pause for 10 seconds on each leg.

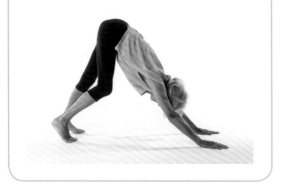

DOWNWARD FACING DOG

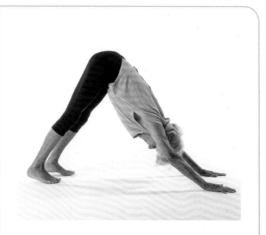

Start on all fours. Spread your fingers wide. Lift your hips up to make a triangle shape with your body. Press both heels down towards the floor.

THREE-LEGGED DOG

Start on all fours. Spread your fingers wide. Lift your hips up to make a triangle shape with your body. Raise your left leg off the floor and press your right heel closer to the floor. Repeat on the other side.

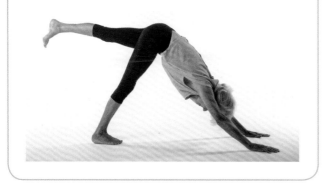

DO THE DOG?

While yoga's Downwards Facing Dog is a fantastic stretch for the calves, it is not suitable for everyone. If you lift your hips up into the position and it feels like a Plank with a ton of weight on your shoulders, arms and wrists, don't struggle. Skip the Dog and choose a non-weight-bearing stretch such as the Standing Toes up Stretch or Step or Block Stretch (see previous page) as these techniques will allow you to focus on the calves in comfort.

Kneeling calf stretches

WINDSCREEN WIPE

Perform a Lunge by starting on all fours and stepping your right foot up between your hands. Shift your body weight back and roll your front foot onto the heel. Point your toes up. 'Windscreen wipe' your foot by swaying it slowly left and right. Repeat on the other side.

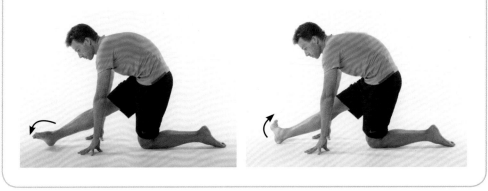

KNEELING CALF STRETCH

Perform a Lunge by starting on all fours and stepping your right foot up between your hands. Shift your body weight back and roll your front foot onto the heel. Point your toes up and/or draw your toes back towards you. To deepen the stretch, hold onto your foot with your right hand and pull gently back.

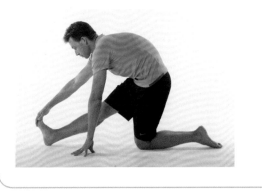

Calf Stretching Tools

If you suffer with tight calf muscles or Achilles, it may be worth investing in a calf-stretching device. The simple 'incline board' device allows you to stand with your feet in a heels down and toes up angle (dorsiflexion). Some are square, solid contraptions made of wood while others feature a rocking design and allow you to control and increase the intensity of the stretch by pressing the heel down or up.

LYING CALF STRAP STRETCH

Lie on your back and loop a strap, belt or tie around the sole of the right foot. Bend the left leg and place the foot on the floor, especially if your hamstrings are tight. Straighten the right leg. Push your heel up. Repeat on the other side.

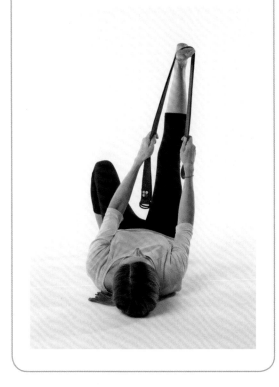

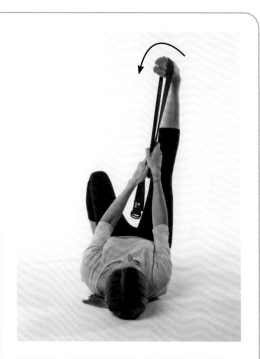

LYING ANKLE STRAP STRETCH

Lie on your back and loop a strap, belt or tie around the sole of the right foot. Bend the left leg and place the foot on the floor, especially if your hamstrings are tight. Straighten the right leg. Turn the sole of your foot to the left. Move your leg 10-20 degrees across your body. Repeat on the other side.

Finding the Achilles

To the untrained eye, one calf stretch looks much like another, but a small adjustment will shift the focus from the upper calves to the lower calves and Achilles tendon. If you have been told to stretch your Achilles, repeat the calf stretches outlined earlier, but bend the back leg. Here are three examples to try:

STANDING ACHILLES STRETCH

Stand with the feet hip-width apart and your hands on your hips. Take a large step back with your left foot, bend your back leg and push your heel down. Bend your right leg a little and push your hips forwards. Repeat on the other side.

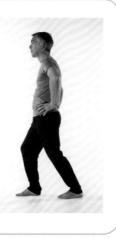

STEP OR BLOCK ACHILLES STRETCH

Stand on the edge of the stairs or a couple of foam yoga blocks or books. Bend both legs a little and drop your left heel off the edge of the platform.

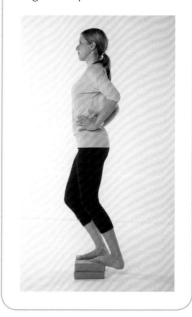

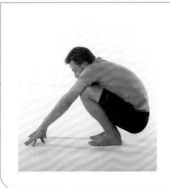

ACHILLES SQUAT STRETCH

Stand with your feet hip-width apart. Bend your legs and lower down into a squatting position with your toes facing forward. Rest your fingertips on the floor in front for balance if necessary.

Stretches for High Heel Wearers

Wearing high heels on a regular basis can shorten the calf muscles and may even cause Achilles tendinitis or inflammation of the Achilles tendon. Try some simple, regular preventative stretches such as the Step or Block Achilles Stretch to reach the calf, remembering to then bend your standing leg to target the Achilles. If you have good foot and ankle flexibility, try the Kneeling Towel Stretch too (page 103).

The Feet and Ankles

This section features a variety of lower limb stretches for all. They will provide relief for those who have been 'on their feet' all day at work, or help runners sidestep foot and ankle injuries caused by pounding the pavements or woodland trails. Techniques range in intensity, from the more challenging kneeling stretches to simply sitting down on a chair, taking your shoes off and 'circling' the feet.

CHAIR FOOT CIRCLES

Sit with your legs bent and feet on the ground. Lift your right foot and rotate it as if drawing circles with your toes. *Repeat x 4.*

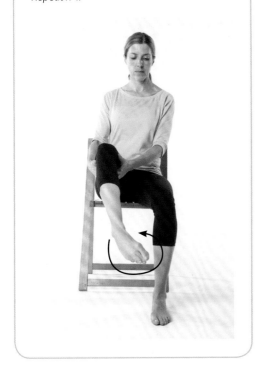

CHAIR POINT AND FLEX

Sit with your legs bent and feet on the ground. Lift your right foot and alternate between pointing your toes and flexing your foot by lifting your toes and pushing your heel forward. *Repeat x 4.*

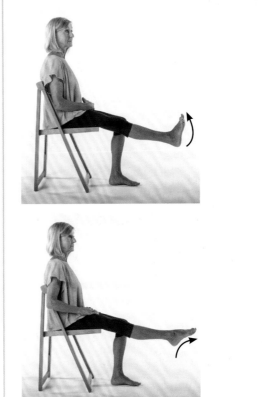

Chair foot stretch sequence

Sit up straight, lift your right foot up and lay the ankle on the left knee.

1 Rotate your foot slowly in circles x 4.

2 Stabilise the foot by holding onto your heel, now:

- Curl your toes in toward the sole
- Pull your toes back to stretch the sole
- Turn the sole of the foot upwards

Repeat on the other side.

A FOOT FLEXIBILITY TEST FOR RUNNERS

Stand with your feet hip-width apart. Reach down and pull your big toe upward. You are aiming for an angle of 30 degrees. If you can't lift this high, your plantar fascia – the layer of connective tissue that connects your toes to the heel and absorbs the shock of walking and running – is too tight. Stretching exercises for the feet, ankles, Achilles and calves are a good preventative measure but self-massage could be the answer. See a physiotherapist for advice.

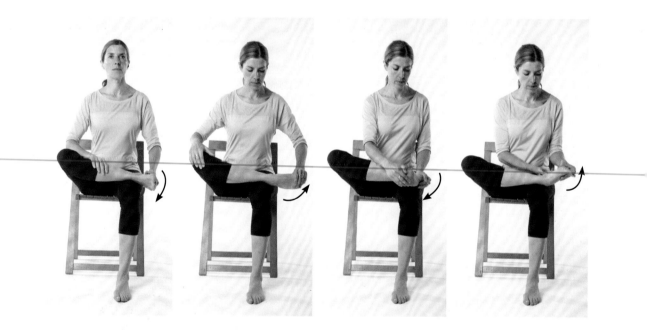

KNEELING

Come to a kneeling position by sitting back onto the heels. This can be made more comfortable if you place three or four cushions between the buttocks and heels, but move in carefully and avoid this kneeling section if there is pain or discomfort.

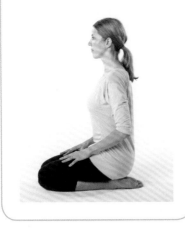

KNEELING SOLE STRETCH

On all fours, turn your toes under to feel a stretch on the soles of the feet. Either remain here or walk your hands backwards until you are sitting back on your heels.

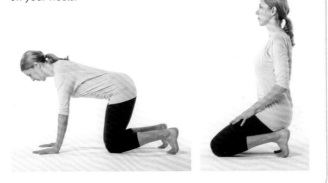

KNEELING TOWEL STRETCH

To gain a deeper stretch for the front of the foot and ankle, perform the kneeling position by sitting back on the heels, but with a small folded towel underneath your toes.

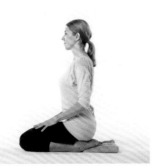

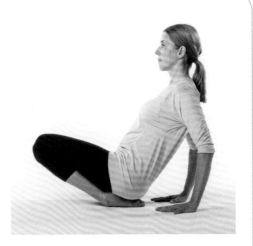

KNEELING SHIN STRETCH

For an advanced front of foot and ankle stretch, come to a kneeling position sitting on your heels. Now lean back and lift your knees off the floor.

Five-minute stretch sequences

String together some stretches into five-minute routines for improved flexibility in the lower leg and foot area.

Lower legs and feet sequence 1

1. ANKLE ROLL

Place your hands on your hips. Stand on your left leg and lift your right foot off the floor. Rotate your foot slowly. *Repeat x 4.*

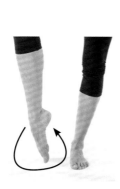

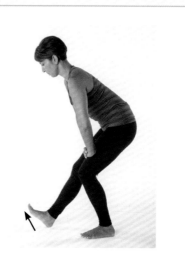

2. STANDING TOES UP STRETCH

Bend your back leg and tip your upper body forwards. Lift your front toes up to roll your foot on the heel. *Hold for 20 seconds.*

3. ACHILLES SQUAT STRETCH

Stand with your feet hip-width apart and your toes facing forwards. Bend your legs and lower down into a squatting position. Rest your fingertips on the floor in front for balance if necessary. *Hold for 30 seconds.*

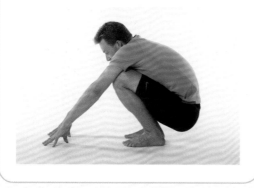

4. WALKING DOG

Start on all fours. Spread your fingers wide. Lift your hips up to make a triangle shape with your body. Bend one leg and push the other heel towards the floor. Continue, moving side to side. *Repeat x 8.*

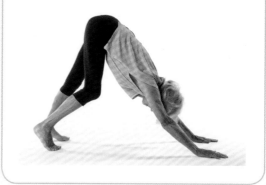

Lower legs and feet sequence 2

CHAIR POINT AND FLEX

Sit on a chair with your legs bent and feet on the ground. Lift your right foot and alternate between pointing your toes and flexing your foot by lifting your toes and pushing your heel forward. Repeat on the other side. *Repeat x 4.*

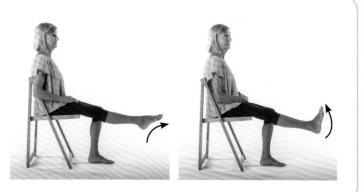

Sit up straight on a chair, lift your right foot up and lay the ankle on the left thigh.

SITTING FOOT STRETCH 1

Rotate your foot slowly in circles. *Repeat x 4.*

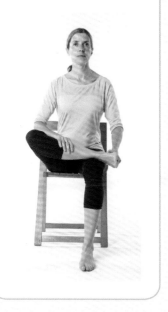

SITTING FOOT STRETCH 2

Curl your toes in towards the sole. *Hold for 10 seconds.*

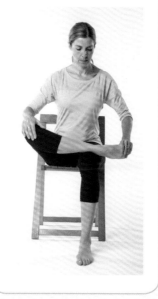

SITTING FOOT STRETCH 3

Pull your toes back to stretch the sole. *Hold for 10 seconds.*

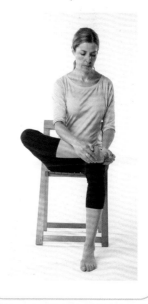

Lower legs and feet sequence 3

1. WINDSCREEN WIPE

Perform a Lunge by starting on all fours and stepping your right foot up between your hands. Shift your body weight back and roll your front foot onto the heel. Point your toes up. 'Windscreen wipe' your foot by swaying it slowly left and right. *Repeat x 6.*

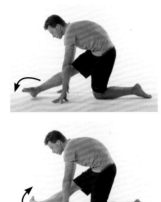

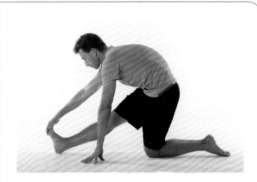

2. KNEELING CALF STRETCH

Perform a Lunge by starting on all fours and stepping your right foot up between your hands. Shift your body weight back and roll your front foot onto the heel. Point your toes up and/or draw your toes back towards you. To deepen the stretch, hold onto your foot with your right hand and pull gently back. *Hold for 20 seconds.* Repeat on the other side.

3. LYING STRAP CALF STRETCH

Lie on your back and loop a strap, belt or tie around the sole of the right foot. Bend the left leg and place the foot on the floor, especially if your hamstrings are tight. Straighten the right leg up towards the ceiling or keep it a little bent. Push your heel up. *Hold for 30 seconds.* Repeat on the other side.

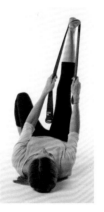

4. LYING ANKLE STRAP STRETCH

Lie on your back and loop a strap, belt or tie around the sole of the right foot. Bend the left leg and place the foot on the floor, especially if your hamstrings are tight. Straighten the right leg up towards the ceiling or keep it a little bent. Turn the sole of your foot to the left. Move your leg 10-20 degrees across your body. *Hold for 30 seconds.* Repeat on the other side.

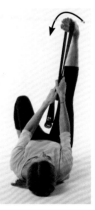

Lower legs and feet sequence 4

1. KNEELING SOLE STRETCH

Start on all fours. Turn your toes under to feel a stretch on the soles of the feet. Either remain here or walk your hands backwards until you are sitting back on your heels. *Hold for 10 seconds.*

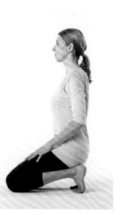

2. KNEELING

Come to a kneeling position by sitting back onto the heels. This can be made more comfortable if you place three or four cushions between the buttocks and heels. *Hold for 20 seconds.*

3. DOWNWARD FACING DOG

Start on all fours. Spread your fingers wide. Lift your hips up to make a triangle shape with your body. Press both heels down towards the floor.

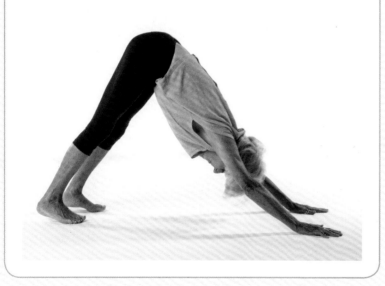

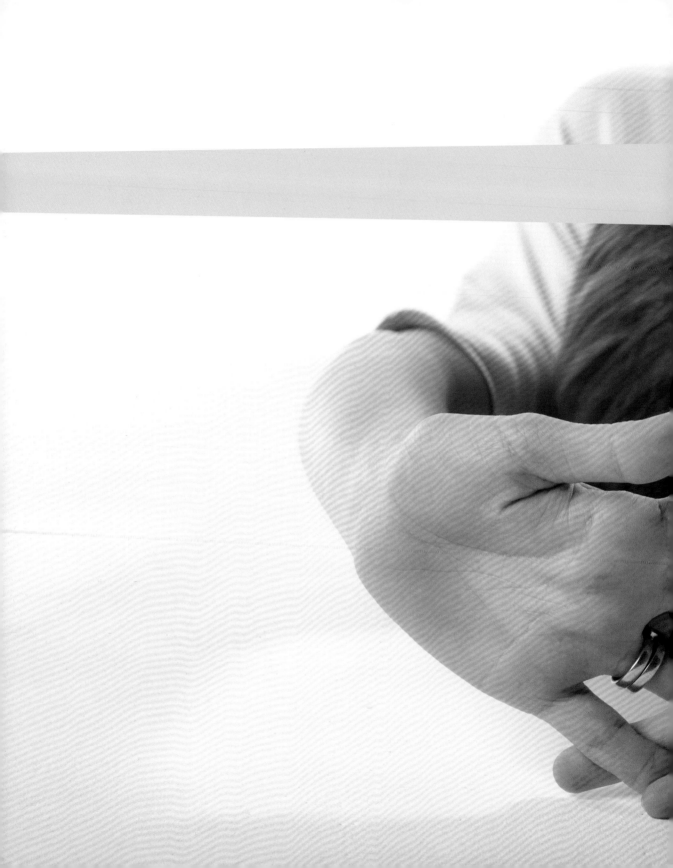

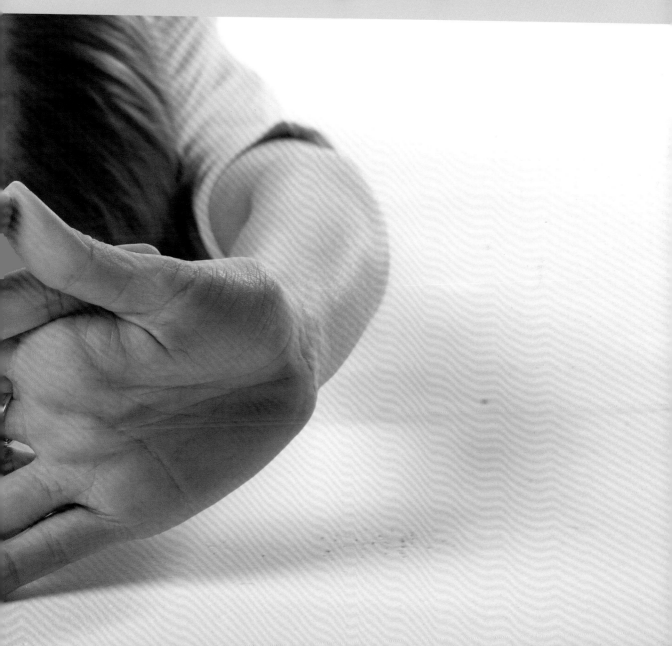

Stretching Sequences

The Morning Wake-Up

Unlock stiff muscles after a long night's sleep and improve circulation with this gentle wake-up sequence. The routine begins lying down in bed by stretching the back so would be ideal for someone prone to lower backache. Then stand or sit on the edge of the bed for the second half of the routine to ease out the upper back, neck and shoulders.

1. LYING FULL BODY STRETCH

Lying down, sweep both arms overhead and interlink your fingers. Turn your palms away. Point your toes to the ceiling. *Hold for 20 seconds.*

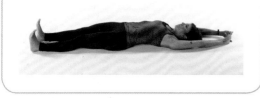

2. SINGLE LEG HUG

Lie on your back and draw your right leg in towards your chest. Keep your left leg straight and press the back of your knee to the bed. Repeat on the other side. *Hold for 20 seconds.*

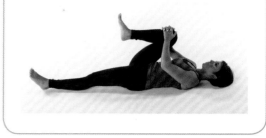

3. DOUBLE LEG HUG

Lie on your back and hug both legs into your abdomen. Rock a little from side to side across your lower back. *Hold for 20 seconds.*

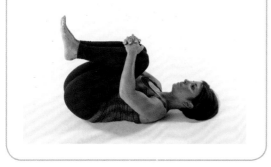

4. BASIC LYING TWIST

Lie on your back. Bend both legs and place your feet flat on the bed (or floor). Stretch your arms out at shoulder height. Lower both legs down to the floor on the left side and relax them. Repeat on the other side. *Hold for 30 seconds.*

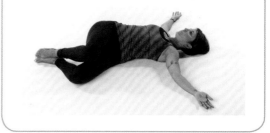

5. DYNAMIC HEAD TURN

Sit on the edge of the bed or stand. Rotate your head to the right, back to the centre and over to the left. Continue to turn your head from side to side. Move in slow motion. *Repeat x 4.*

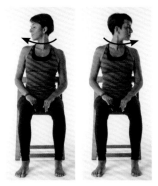

6. SHOULDER BLADE SQUEEZE

Hold your arms in a 'W' shape. Draw them back and squeeze your shoulder blades together. Release and bring your forearms closer or touching. *Repeat x 4.*

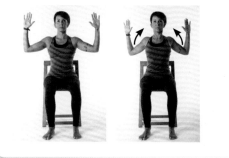

7. CLASPED HANDS NECK STRETCH

Take your hands behind your back. Interlink them and slide them around the right side of your waist. Tip your head over to the right. *Hold for 20 seconds.*

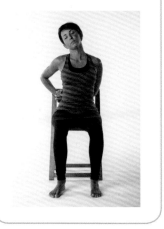

8. STANDING OR SITTING SIDE BEND

Sit or stand tall and lean to the side, aiming not to tip forwards or back. To go deeper, try clasping the top wrist and side bending further. *Hold for 10 seconds.*

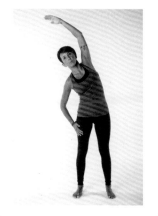

9. FULL BODY SIDE BEND

Stand with your feet hip-width apart. Sweep your arms up overhead and interlink your fingers. Now lean to the side aiming not to tip forwards or backwards. To go deeper, try clasping the top wrist and side bending further. Repeat on the other side. *Hold for 20 seconds.*

The Commuter

If you spend at least two hours a day driving your car, or travelling on trains or buses to and from work, or are a frequent flyer, here is a sequence to ease the stiffening effects of the sedentary commute. They are all small, subtle movements that can be done without drawing attention from fellow commuters.

1. THE CHIN TUCK

Tuck your chin into your chest as if nodding but hold the stretch. *Hold for 10 seconds.*

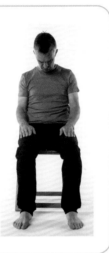

2. DYNAMIC HEAD TURN

Rotate your head to the right, back to the centre and over to the left. Continue to turn your head from side to side. Move in slow motion. *Repeat x 4.*

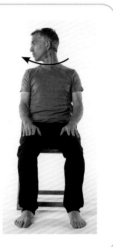

3. DYNAMIC HEAD TILT

Tip your right ear down towards your right shoulder. Return to the centre. Tip your left ear down towards your left shoulder. Return to the centre. Continue to tilt your head from side to side slowly and smoothly. *Repeat x 4.*

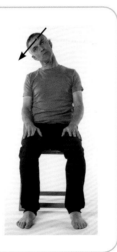

4. SHOULDER SHRUG

Lift your shoulders up towards your ears. Hold for a second. Now let them drop down. *Repeat x 4.*

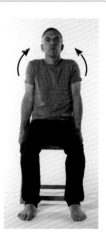

5. CHAIR SEATED TWIST

Sit tall. Hold onto the left side of your chair and rotate your torso to the left in sections: lower back, mid back and shoulders and finally turn your head. Repeat on the other side. *Hold for 10 seconds*

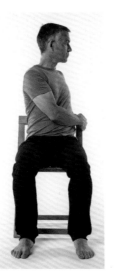

6. SQUEEZE AND SPREAD

Squeeze your hands into fists tucking the thumb in and hold for five seconds. Now spread your hands wide and hold for five seconds. *Repeat x 4.*

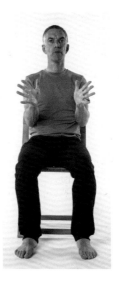

7. CHAIR FOOT CIRCLE

Sit with your legs bent and feet on the ground. Lift your right foot and rotate it as if drawing circles with your toes. Repeat on the other side. *Repeat x 4.*

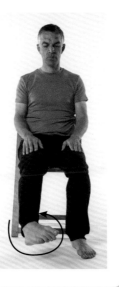

8. CHAIR POINT AND FLEX

Sit with your legs bent and feet on the ground. Lift your right foot and alternate between pointing your toes and flexing your foot (by pushing your heel forward). *Repeat x 4.*

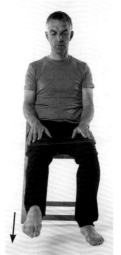

The Desk Worker

Offset time spent sitting at your desk with this routine, designed to relieve wrist, neck and back tension and unlock the hips. The seated position can be particularly tough on the lower back. A few simple movements such as stretching the arms overhead and holding (Chair Back Stretch) can also wake up the body and mind and allow you to continue working with renewed energy. Regular walking breaks around the office every 20 minutes are also recommended by physical therapists as well as ensuring that your work station is set up for maximum comfort and minimum strain

1. WRIST AND HAND WARMER

Sitting on a chair, interlace your fingers, palms down and chest-height. Pull your hands slightly apart as if your fingers were stuck together until you can feel some traction. Then, alternately flex and extend (bend and draw back) your wrists. *Repeat x 4.*

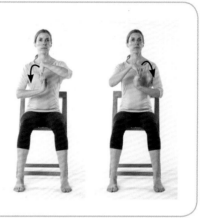

2. CHAIR BACK STRETCH

Sit tall. Sweep your arms up overhead and interlink your fingers. Press your palms towards the ceiling and remain here, drawing your shoulders downwards. *Hold for 10 seconds.*

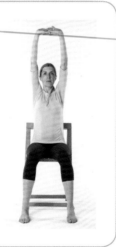

3. CHAIR SIDE BEND

From the Chair Back Stretch position, simply lean to the side aiming not to tip forwards or backwards. To go deeper, try clasping your top wrist and side bending further. *Hold for 20 seconds.*

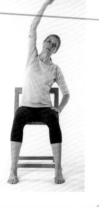

4. CHAIR CAT STRETCH

Sit tall. Rest your hands lightly on your thighs. As you inhale, arch your back and look a little upwards. As you exhale, round your back and tuck your pelvis and chin in. *Repeat x 4.*

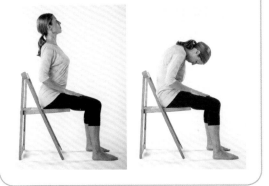

5. CHAIR SEATED TWIST

Sit tall. Hold onto the right side of your chair and rotate your torso to the right in sections: lower back, mid back and shoulders, and finally turn your head. *Hold for 20 seconds.*

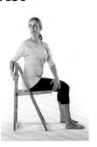

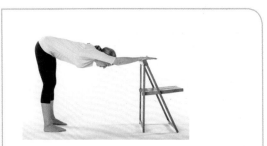

6. FIGURE FOUR CHAIR

Sit with a straight back and both feet on the ground. Lift your left foot off the floor and turn your knee out. Rest your left ankle on top of your right thigh. Keeping the back straight, lean the upper body forwards. Lean further to increase the intensity of the stretch. Repeat on the other side. *Hold for 30 seconds.*

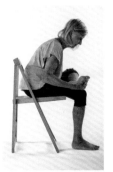

7. 90-DEGREE CHAIR STRETCH

Stand behind a chair and place your hands on the top of the chair back, shoulder-width apart. Walk backwards until you fold into a 90-degree position. Move your head in line with the spine. To exit, walk forwards, bend your knees and rise up to a standing position. *Hold for 30 seconds.*

8. CHAIR HIGH LUNGE

Stand in front of a chair with your hands on your hips. Place your right foot on the chair seat and bend your right leg. Push your hips forwards. Repeat on the other side. *Hold for 20 seconds.*

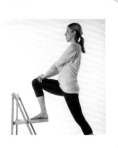

The Manual Worker

This short sequence done daily will release muscles tired and tight from a physical day's work, especially around the back, neck and shoulder regions. If you are short on time or lack the energy for the entire routine, pay particular attention to your lower back stretches (Single Leg Hug and Basic Lying Twist), both of which can be done lying in bed, as it is important to look after your lower back if repeatedly bending or lifting heavy loads.

1. WRIST ROLL

Make fists with both hands and rotate them slowly. *Repeat x 4.*

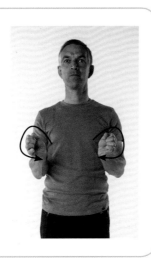

2. FULL BODY STRETCH

Stand with your feet hip-width apart. Sweep your arms up overhead and interlink your fingers. Press your palms towards the ceiling and remain here, drawing your shoulders downwards. *Hold for 10 seconds.*

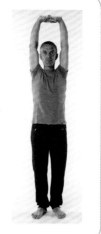

3. FULL BODY SIDE BEND

From the Full Body Stretch position, simply lean to the side aiming not to tip forwards or backwards. To go deeper, try clasping the top wrist and side bending further. *Hold for 20 seconds.*

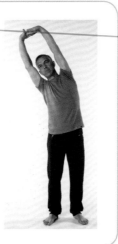

4. ASSISTED NECK EXTENSOR STRETCH

Stand or sit tall. Interlink your hands behind your head. Drop your head down, bringing your chin towards your chest. Do not push your head further, but let your elbows drop forwards so that the weight of your arms increases the stretch. *Hold for 10 seconds.*

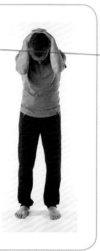

5. CHEST AND SHOULDER STRETCH

Take your arms behind your back and interlink your hands. Lift your chest, draw your shoulders back and raise your hands. Lift your hands higher, without leaning forward, to go deeper. *Hold for 20 seconds.*

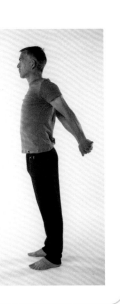

6. LEAN FORWARD STRETCH

Take a small step back with your left leg. Bend your left leg and tip your upper body forwards, placing both hands on your right thigh. Press the sole of the right foot into the floor. Repeat on the other side. *Hold for 20 seconds.*

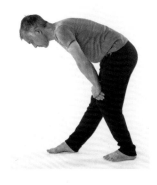

7. SINGLE LEG HUG

Lie on your back and draw your right leg in towards your chest. Keep your left leg straight and press the back of the left knee into the floor. *Hold for 20 seconds.*

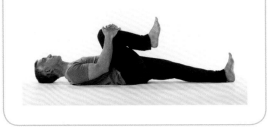

8. BASIC LYING TWIST

Lie on your back. Bend both legs and place your feet on the floor. Stretch your arms out at shoulder height. Lower both legs down to the floor on the left side and relax them. *Hold for 30 seconds.*

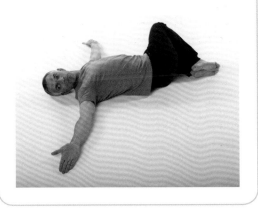

Four Time-Pressed Routines

Can't find the time to stretch? You are not alone! Sometimes all you have is a few moments to spare. Here are four rapid sequences to loosen up the whole body and maintain overall flexibility which take three to five minutes each. They are split into Standing, Seated, Floor and Lying stretches, but you can slot the sequences together to create a longer 10, 15 or 20-minute routine if you find more time.

Standing

1. FULL BODY STRETCH

Stand with your feet hip-width apart. Sweep your arms up overhead and interlink your fingers. Press your palms towards the ceiling and remain here, drawing your shoulders downwards. *Hold for 10 seconds.*

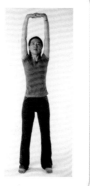

2. FULL BODY SIDE BEND

From the Full Body Stretch position, simply lean to the side aiming not to tip forwards or backwards. To go deeper try clasping the top wrist and side bending further. *Hold for 20 seconds.*

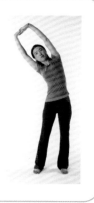

3. STANDING BACK BEND

Place your hands on your lower back, fingers pointing downwards. Lean back into a gentle backbend and push your hips forwards. Draw your elbows together. *Hold for 10 seconds.*

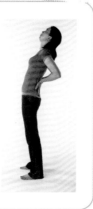

4. 90-DEGREE STRETCH

Tip your upper body forwards until you reach a 90-degree angle, or higher. Do not allow the back to curve. Draw the abdomen slightly inwards. Place your hand on your calves, just below your knees. *Hold for 20 seconds.*

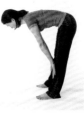

Seated

1. CHAIR CAT STRETCH

Rest your hands lightly on your thighs. As you inhale, arch your back and look a little upwards. As you exhale, round your back and tuck your pelvis and chin in. *Repeat x 4.*

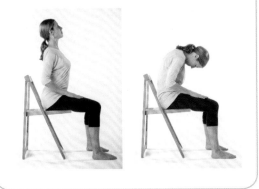

2. CHAIR SEATED TWIST

Sit tall. Hold onto the right side of your chair and rotate your torso to the right in sections: lower back, mid back and shoulders and finally turn your head. *Hold for 20 seconds.*

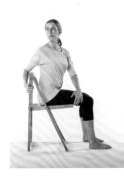

3. FIGURE FOUR CHAIR

Sit on a chair with a straight back and both feet on the floor. Lift your left foot off the floor and turn your knee out. Rest your left ankle on top of your right thigh. Keeping the back straight, lean the upper body forwards. Lean further to increase the intensity of the stretch. *Hold for 20 seconds.*

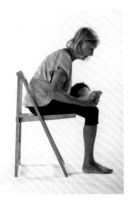

4. CHAIR FORWARD BEND

Let your back round and head drop down. If the back feels very stiff, rest your hands on your thighs or lean further forwards until your hands touch the floor. *Hold for 30 seconds.*

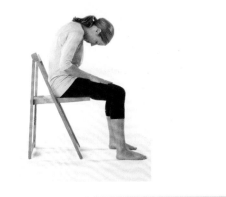

Floor

1. LOW LUNGE

Lower yourself down to all fours. Step your right foot up in between your hands and raise the upper body. Push your hips forwards. Slowly sink the hips forwards and down into the lunge. Repeat on the other side. *Hold for 30 seconds.*

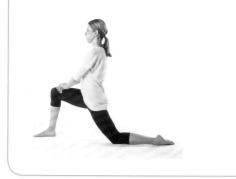

2. KNEELING CALF STRETCH

Shift your body weight back and roll your front foot onto the heel. Point your toes up and/or draw your toes back towards you. Repeat on the other side. *Hold for 20 seconds.*

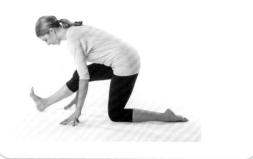

3. BUTTERFLY

Sit with a straight back, perching on the edge of a cushion or two if this makes it more comfortable. Bring the soles of your feet together. Either clasp your hands around the feet or hold onto your ankles and sit taller. *Hold for 30 seconds.*

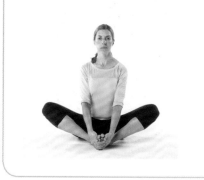

4. BASIC SEATED TWIST

Sit with your legs out straight. Bend your left leg and step it over your right. Wrap your right arm around your leg and hug your leg into your body. Drop your left fingertips onto the floor behind your back and begin to rotate the torso to the left in stages: lower back, mid back and shoulders, and head. Repeat on the other side. *Hold for 30 seconds.*

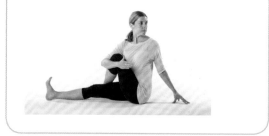

Lying

1. SINGLE LEG HUG

Lie on your back and draw your right leg in towards your chest. Keep your left leg straight and press the back of the left knee into the floor. Repeat on the other side. *Hold for 20 seconds.*

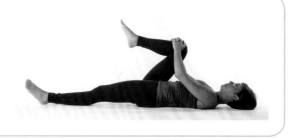

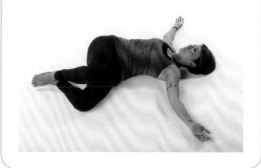

2. SIDE LYING QUAD STRETCH

Lie on your left side with your left leg a little bent under you for balance. Bend your right leg and reach for the foot. Push your hips forward. Repeat on the other side. *Hold for 20 seconds.*

3. LYING HAMSTRING STRAP STRETCH

Lie on your back and loop a strap, belt or tie around the sole of your right foot. Bend your left leg and place your foot on the floor, especially if your hamstrings are tight. Straighten your right leg or keep it a little bent. Repeat on the other side. *Hold for 30 seconds.*

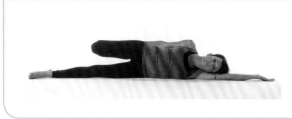

4. BASIC LYING TWIST

Bend both legs and place your feet on the floor. Stretch your arms out at shoulder height. Lower both legs down the floor on the left side and relax them. *Hold for 30 seconds.*

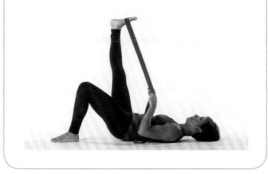

Better Posture Sequence

Standing or sitting taller is not only the healthiest way to position your muscles and joints, it also reduces muscular strain, particularly on the lower back, provides a psychological confidence boost (just sit up straight and see), and improves breathing efficiency. Modern life demands that we sit a lot while driving, commuting, working at the office or relaxing on the sofa, and the temptation to slouch is ever present, so draw your shoulders back and lengthen the spine with the following sequence.

Have an old tie or dressing gown belt handy for steps 1 and 2.

1. STRAP SHOULDER LOOSENER

Hold a strap or tie overhead with your hands wide apart and play with the following movements:

1. Drop your hands forwards so the strap is in front of your chest.

2. Lift the strap overhead so it is behind your head. *Repeat x 4.*

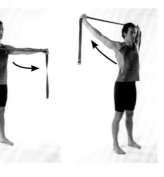

2. OVERHEAD STRAP STRETCH

Remain standing. Raise your strap, tie or belt overhead with your hands wide. Bend your arms until they form a 90-degree angle and draw your elbows back. *Hold for 20 seconds.*

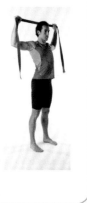

3. CHEST AND SHOULDER STRETCH

Take your arms behind your back and interlink your hands. Lift your chest, draw your shoulders back and raise your hands. Do not lean forward. Lift your hands higher to go deeper. *Hold for 20 seconds.*

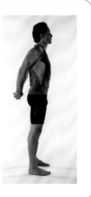

4. WAITER'S BOW

Stand with your feet hip-width apart. Place your right hand on the dip of your lower back, palm facing outward. Place your left palm on your abdomen. Keeping your lower back curve intact, tip forwards. Stop when your back begins to round. *Hold for 20 seconds.*

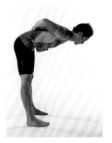

5. LOW LUNGE

Lower yourself down to all fours. Step your right foot up in between your hands and raise your upper body. Push your hips forward. Slowly lower into the lunge. Repeat on the other side. *Hold for 30 seconds.*

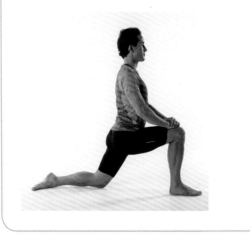

6. SNAKE

Lie on your front with your hands interlocked behind your back (or arms straight by your sides). Draw your shoulder blades closer and lift your upper body and legs a little off the floor. Look down, not forwards. *Hold for 20 seconds.*

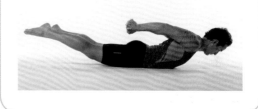

7. KNEELING BACK STRETCH

Lift back to all fours. Sit back on your heels. Straighten your arms and reach your hands to the top of your mat. Spread your fingers and press down. Draw your hips away in the opposite direction to stretch your shoulders and back. *Hold for 20 seconds.*

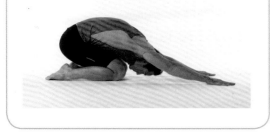

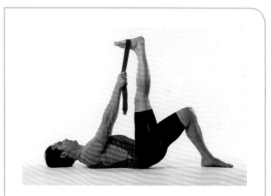

8. LYING HAMSTRING STRAP STRETCH

Lie on your back and loop a strap, belt or tie around the sole of your right foot. Bend your left leg and place the foot on the floor, especially if your hamstrings are tight. Straighten your right leg or keep it a little bent. Repeat on the other side. *Hold for 30 seconds.*

Stretches for Children

Younger children often stretch spontaneously by flipping upside down, twisting or practising the latest gymnastics moves from school. However, I noticed a dramatic decrease in my children's levels of hip and hamstring flexibility particularly when they transitioned from regularly sitting cross-legged in assemblies and the classroom to using chairs. By making stretching fun, children can maintain that enviable flexibility and create the habit of a lifetime. I have recommended holding most stretches for only ten seconds with plenty of rocking and rolling to account for short attention spans, but the entire sequence could be repeated two or three times if it feels too short.

1. BANANA

Lie on your back. Sweep your arms overhead, clasp your hands together and move your hands and feet over to the left so that your body bends like a banana. Bend to the other side. *Hold for 10 seconds.*

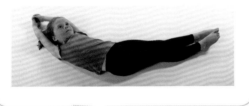

2. PENCIL

Keep your arms overhead but bring your palms together. Point your toes. *Hold for 10 seconds.*

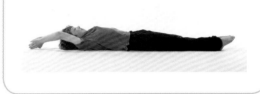

3. DISH

From Pencil, keep your arms above your head and roll onto your tummy. Sweep your arms by your side and lift your feet off the floor. *Hold for 10 seconds.*

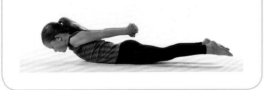

4. THE LEG PULL

Roll onto your right side and balance here. Bend your top leg, hold your foot and pull the leg back while pushing your hips forward. Roll onto your other side and repeat. *Hold for 10 seconds.*

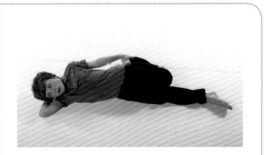

5. ROLLING BALL

Return to lying on your back. Hug your legs into your body tightly and rock from side to side. *Repeat x 4.*

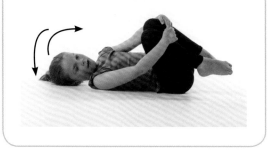

6. SOCK STRETCH

Lie on your back. Take a sock off and loop it around your right foot. Bend your left leg and put your left foot on the floor. Straighten your right leg but keep a small bend in your knee. Repeat on the other side. *Hold for 10 seconds.*

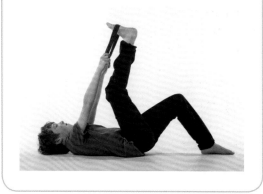

7. TWIST

Stretch your arms out to the sides. Bend your legs and put your feet on the floor. Now drop both knees over to the left side and turn your head to the right. Repeat on the other side. *Hold for 10 seconds.*

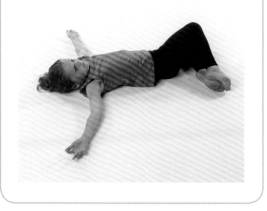

8. BUTTERFLY

Sit up. Bring the soles of your feet together. Clasp your hands around your feet and sit tall. *Hold for 10 seconds.*

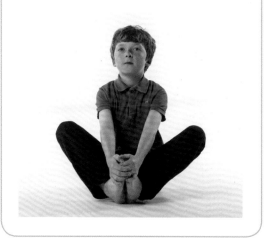

Stretches for Teenagers

Teenagers don't always have the time or inclination to stretch, but this short routine will release tight muscles after athletic endeavours, improve mood and posture, and reduce exam stress. Teenagers also spend large amounts of time sitting at school or college. This, combined with the heavy use of electronic devices, causes tension in the neck and spine, and stretching can address this. Remember, never push a stretch to the point of pain or use jerky movements to bounce the body in and out of stretches. After performing the warm-up moves (steps 1-4), hold each stretch still and breathe slowly through your nose.

1. HEAD ROLL

Make a continuous semi-circle movement with your head by first tipping your head to the right side by dropping your ear to your shoulder, looking down at your feet, then rolling your head around to the left shoulder. Move in slow motion. Don't tip your head back. Repeat in the other direction. *Repeat x 4.*

2. ELBOW TOUCH

Drop your fingertips onto your shoulders. Sit or stand tall. Breathe in as you draw your elbows wide. Breathe out as you draw your elbows closer or together. *Repeat x 4.*

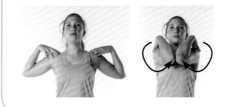

3. SQUEEZE AND SPREAD

Squeeze your hands into fists tucking the thumb in and hold for five seconds. Now spread your hands wide and hold for five seconds. *Repeat x 4.*

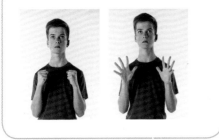

4. DYNAMIC SIDE BENDING

Stand with your feet hip-width apart. Sweep your left arm up and tip over to the right, trying not to lean forwards or backwards. Return to the centre. Sweep the right arm up and tip to the left. *Repeat x 4.*

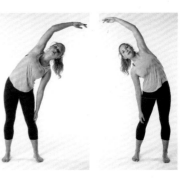

5. CHEST AND SHOULDER STRETCH

Take your arms behind your back and interlink your hands. Lift your chest, draw your shoulders back and raise your hands. Lift your hands higher, without leaning forward, to go deeper. *Hold for 20 seconds.*

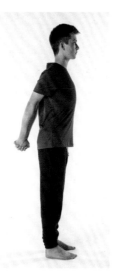

6. FULL FORWARD BEND

Stand with your feet hip-width apart. Bend your knees a little. Fold forward and let your upper body hang. Relax your head and let your arms dangle. *Hold for 60 seconds.* Uncurl slowly up to standing.

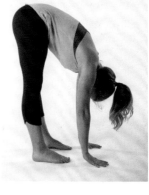

7. LOW LUNGE

Lower yourself down to all fours. Step your right foot up in between your hands and raise your upper body. Push your hips forward. Slowly lower into the lunge. *Hold for 30 seconds.*

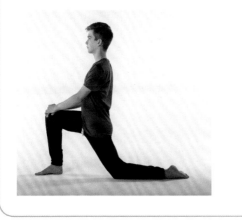

8. TORTOISE

Sit with your legs in a diamond shape and the soles of your feet together. Let your upper body drop forwards so your back rounds and your head hangs down. Rest your forearms on your legs or hold onto your feet. *Hold for 30 seconds.*

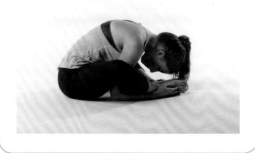

Stretches for Seniors

It's impossible to make assumptions about people's flexibility or strength levels based on their age. I have clients that have practised yoga and Pilates for 20 years and could happily do the *Total Body Flexibility: Advanced Sequences* (see page 144). However, most people find themselves becoming stiffer as they age and move less. A little regular stretching can offset this decline in mobility as well as improving posture and breathing. A few safety notes: talk with your doctor if you are unsure about a particular technique, especially if you have had hip or back surgery, never stretch to the point of discomfort, and avoid 'locking' your joints by keeping your legs slightly bent while stretching.

1. CHAIR FOOT CIRCLE

Sit with your legs bent and feet on the ground. Lift your right foot and rotate it as if drawing circles with your toes. Repeat on the other side. *Repeat x 4.*

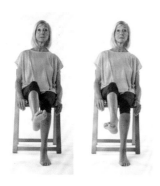

2. CHAIR POINT AND FLEX

Sit with your legs bent and feet on the ground. Lift your right foot and alternate between pointing your toes and flexing your foot (lifting your toes and pushing your heel forward). Repeat on the other side. *Repeat x 4.*

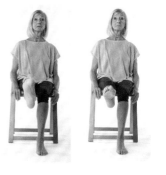

3. CHAIR SIDE BEND

Sit tall and lean to your right side. To go deeper try clasping the top wrist and side bending further. Repeat on the other side. *Hold for 10 seconds.*

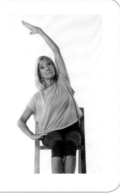

4. CHAIR SEATED TWIST

Hold onto the left side of your chair and rotate your torso to the left in sections: lower back, mid back and shoulders and your head. Repeat on the other side. *Hold for 20 seconds.*

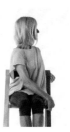

5. 90-DEGREE CHAIR STRETCH

Stand behind the chair and place your hands on the top of the chair, shoulder-width apart. Walk back until you fold forward. Try not to round your back. To exit, walk forwards, bend your knees, draw your abdomen in and rise up to standing. *Hold for 20 seconds.*

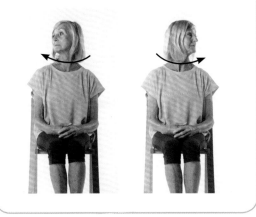

6. CHAIR CALF STRETCH

Stay behind the chair. Step your left leg forward and bend your knee. Bend your right knee slightly, but keep the soles of both feet on the floor.

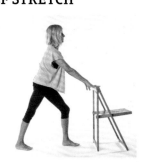

Repeat on the other side. *Hold for 20 seconds.*

7. DYNAMIC HEAD TURN

Rotate your head to the right, back to the centre and over to the left. Continue to turn your head from side to side. Move in slow motion. *Repeat x 4.*

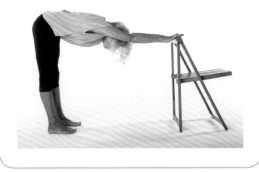

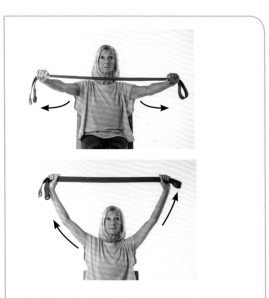

8. STRAP SHOULDER LOOSENER

Hold a strap or tie with your hands wide apart and play with the following movements:

1. Drop your hands forwards so the strap is in front of your chest.

2. Lift the strap overhead so it is behind your head. *Repeat x 4.*

Eight Stretches with a Strap

This sequence would suit anyone who struggles to touch their toes, but wants to experience the same range of stretches as the more mobile. A simple strap, in the form of a cotton yoga strap, dressing gown belt or tie, will expand your range of motion and allow you to stretch without straining the lower back particularly. Everyone, regardless of flexibility levels, can benefit from using a strap when stretching the upper body. The Overhead Strap Stretch accesses tight chest and shoulder muscles hard to reach without a stretching aid and is a great posture improver.

1. OVERHEAD STRAP STRETCH

Stand with your feet hip-width apart. Raise your strap, tie or belt overhead with your hands wide. Bend your arms until they form a 90-degree angle and draw your elbows back. *Hold for 20 seconds.*

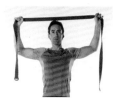

2. ADVANCED TRICEPS STRETCH WITH STRAP

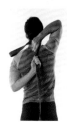

Remain standing. Lay a strap, belt or tie over your left shoulder. Reach up with your right arm and bend it so your hand drops behind your upper back. Take your left arm behind your back and slide it up the spine. Use the strap to bridge the gap between your hands. *Hold for 20 seconds.*

3. SEATED HAMSTRING AND HIP STRAP STRETCH

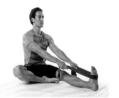

Bend your right leg and place the sole of your foot into your inner left thigh. Sit up straight and loop the strap around the left foot. Remain upright or tilt your upper body forwards without rounding your back. Repeat on the other side. *Hold for 30 seconds.*

4. LYING QUAD STRAP STRETCH

Loop the strap around your right foot. Lower down onto your front. Press your hips into the floor and draw the leg closer to your buttocks. Repeat on the other side. Note: discard the strap if you can comfortably hold the foot. *Hold for 20 seconds.*

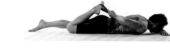

5. LYING HAMSTRING STRAP STRETCH

Lie on your back and loop the strap around the sole of your right foot. Bend your left leg and place your foot on the floor, especially if your hamstrings are tight. Straighten your right leg up towards the ceiling or keep it a little bent. *Hold for 30 seconds.*

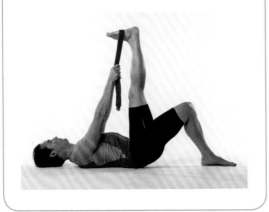

6. LYING CALF STRAP STRETCH

Remain in the Lying Strap Hamstring Stretch position, but move your strap higher onto the ball of the foot. Push your heel up for a deeper stretch. Repeat on the other side. *Hold for 20 seconds.*

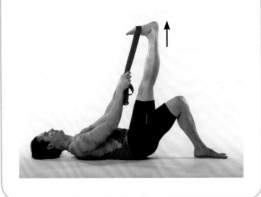

7. LYING INNER THIGH STRAP STRETCH

Stay with your right leg elevated. Hold both parts of your strap in your right hand. Bend your left leg and let your knee drop out to the side. Now slowly take the right leg out to the right. Repeat on the other side.

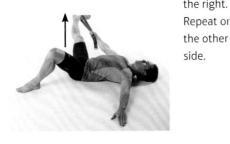

8. LYING OUTER THIGH STRAP STRETCH

Draw your right leg back to the centre and hold both parts of the strap in your left hand. Slide your left leg down and stretch your right arm out along the floor. Begin to take your right leg slowly across to the left. Repeat on the other side. *Hold for 30 seconds.*

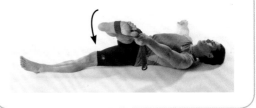

The Stress Reducer

Stretching is a quick and effective way to release stress. The routine below can be performed while sitting at a desk and features a mixture of 'squeeze and release' techniques to shed muscular tension, and longer-held static stretches to slow the heart rate. Most target the fast-twitch muscles of the neck and upper back, which can easily tense up under pressure. Pick two or three techniques or run through the whole sequence remembering to breathe slowly, ideally through your nose.

1. SQUEEZE AND SPREAD

Squeeze your hands into fists tucking the thumb in and hold for five seconds. Now spread your hands wide and hold for five seconds. *Repeat x 4.*

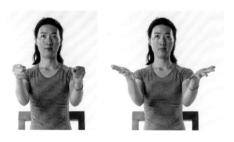

2. HEAD ROLL

Make a continuous semi-circle movement with your head by first tipping your head to the right side (ear to shoulder), rolling it down so you are looking at the floor, then around to the left shoulder. Move in slow motion. Don't tip your head back. Repeat in the other direction. *Repeat x 4.*

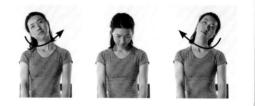

3. ASSISTED NECK EXTENSOR STRETCH

Stand or sit tall. Interlink your hands behind your head. Drop your head down, bringing your chin towards your chest. Do not push your head further, but let your elbows drop forwards so that the weight of your arms increases the stretch. *Hold for 10 seconds.*

4. SHOULDER ROLL

Drop your fingertips onto your shoulders and 'swim' your arms by making alternate circles with your elbows. Roll your shoulders first forwards, then in a backwards motion. *Repeat x 4.*

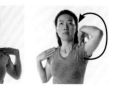

5. SHOULDER SHRUG

Lift your shoulders up towards your ears.
Hold for a second. Now let them drop down.
Repeat x 4.

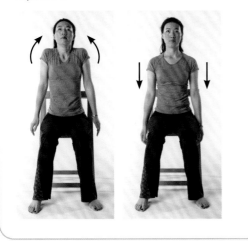

6. STANDING UPPER BACK ROUNDER

Stand with your feet hip-width apart. Round your upper back and tuck your chin in. Reach both arms forwards and interlock your fingers. *Hold for 10 seconds.*

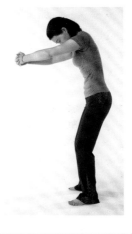

7. CHAIR TWIST

Sit tall. Hold onto the left side of your chair and rotate your torso to the left in sections: lower back, mid back and shoulders and finally turn your head. *Hold for 20 seconds.*

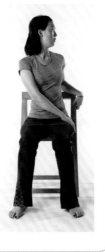

8. CHAIR FORWARD BEND

Round your back and let your head drop downwards. If your back feels very stiff, rest your hands on your thighs or lean further forwards until your hands touch the floor. *Hold for 20 seconds.*

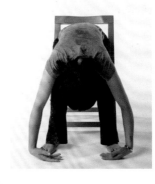

The Pre-Bed Relaxer

Have trouble winding down after a tough day or suffer with insomnia? A regular routine of longer-held stretches may help, especially if combined with deep breathing. The techniques outlined below are 'passive' stretches, meaning that they require no strength or balance. Some are held for a minute to encourage muscle relaxation. Breathe through your nose and perform the moving stretches in slow motion. Once you are familiar with the sequence, perform it with your eyes closed.

1. SLOW ROLL DOWN

Stand with a slight bend in your knees. Drop your head down, lean a little forward and let your arms dangle. Start to roll down in slow motion by letting your upper back, then mid back round. Take four or five slow breaths (one breath = an inhalation and an exhalation) to perform the Slow Roll Down.

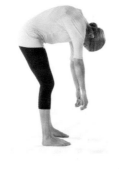

2. CAT STRETCH

Start on all fours. As you inhale, lift your head and hips, allowing your mid back to dip. As you exhale, tuck the chin and hips under allowing your back to round. *Repeat x 4.*

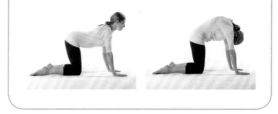

3. CHILD'S POSE

From all fours, lower yourself slowly down to sit on your heels. Rest your forehead on the floor and relax your arms by your sides. If your forehead does not reach the floor, place some foam blocks or cushions under your forehead to raise the floor level. *Hold for 60 seconds.*

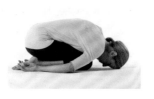

4. KNEELING BACK STRETCH

From all fours, lower yourself down to sit on your heels. Straighten your arms and reach your hands out in front of you. Spread your fingers and press down. Now draw your hips away in the opposite direction. *Hold for 60 seconds.*

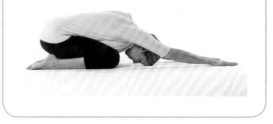

5. BASIC SEATED TWIST

Sit with your legs out straight. Bend your right leg and step it over your left. Wrap your left arm around your leg and hug your leg into your body. Drop your right fingertips onto the floor behind your back and begin to rotate the torso to the right in stages: lower back, mid back and shoulders, and head. Repeat on the other side. *Hold for 20 seconds.*

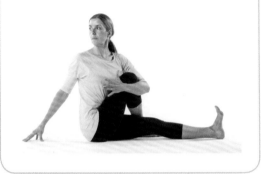

6. DIAMOND

Sit with a straight back, perching on the edge of a cushion or two if this makes it more comfortable. Bring the soles of your feet together, but move them further away until the legs form a diamond shape. Keep your back straight and lean your upper body forwards. *Hold for 60 seconds.*

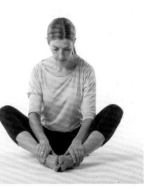

7. TORTOISE

Perform Diamond, but this time allow your back to round and let your head drop downwards. Rest your forearms on your legs or slide them under your legs and hold onto your feet. *Hold for 60 seconds.*

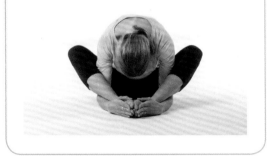

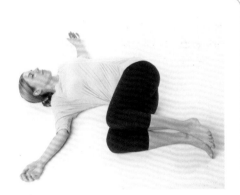

8. BASIC LYING TWIST

Bend both legs and place your feet on the floor. Stretch your arms out at shoulder height, palms facing upwards. Lower both legs down to the floor on the right side and relax them. Repeat on the other side. *Hold for 60 seconds.*

Total Body Flexibility: Gentle Sequences

These stretches are designed either for those who might deem themselves 'stiff' in terms of flexibility, be older in years, or recovering from illness or an operation and are keen to regain mobility in a gentle way. As with all stretching, a low-level activity to raise the heart rate, such as walking, prepares the body for stretching. Raise your body temperature before beginning any of the three routines by simply walking or marching on the spot and rolling your shoulders.

Sequence 1

1. POSTERIOR SHOULDER STRETCH

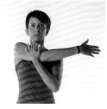

Stand with your right arm straight and at chest height. Place your left hand behind your right elbow and draw your arm across your body. Do not rotate the torso. Repeat on the other side. *Hold for 10 seconds.*

2. TRICEPS STRETCH

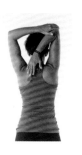

Reach up with your right arm and bend it so your hand drops behind your upper back. Use your left hand to gently draw your right elbow back. Repeat on the other side. *Hold for 10 seconds.*

3. STANDING TOES UP STRETCH

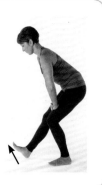

Take a step back with your left leg. Bend your left leg and tip your upper body forwards. Lift your right toes up to roll your foot on your heel. Repeat on the other side. *Hold for 20 seconds.*

4. HIGH LUNGE

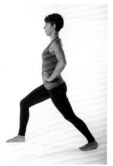

Stand with your feet hip-width apart and your hands on your hips. Take a large step back with your left foot and press your back heel down. Bend your left knee a little and push your hips forwards. *Hold for 20 seconds.*

5. CAT STRETCH

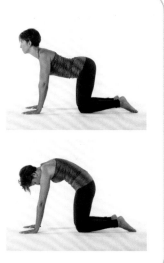

Start from all fours. As you inhale, lift your head and hips, allowing the mid back to dip. As you exhale, tuck the chin and hips under allowing your back to round. *Repeat x 4.*

6. SEATED LEG HUG

Sit with your legs out straight. Bend your right leg and step it over your left. Wrap both arms around your leg and hug it into your body. Sit up straight. Repeat on the other side. *Hold for 20 seconds.*

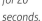
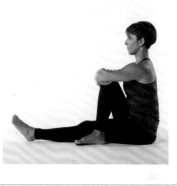

7. BASIC LYING TWIST

Lie on your back. Bend both legs and place your feet on the floor. Stretch your arms out shoulder-height, palms facing upwards. Lower both legs down to the floor on the left side and relax them. Repeat on the other side. *Hold for 30 seconds.*

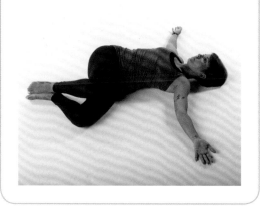

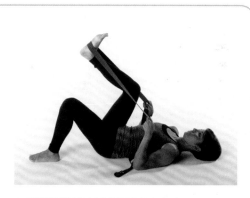

8. LYING HAMSTRING STRAP STRETCH WITH BENT LEG

Lie on your back and loop a strap, belt or tie around the sole of your right foot. Bend your left leg and place your foot on the floor. Raise your right leg up, but keep your leg a little bent. Work on gradually straightening the leg over time. Repeat on the other side. *Hold for 30 seconds.*

Sequence 2

1. HEAD ROLL

Make a continuous semi-circle movement with your head by first tipping your head to the right side by dropping your ear to your shoulder, looking down at your feet, then rolling your head around to the left shoulder. Move in slow motion. Don't tip your head back. Repeat in the other direction. *Repeat x 4.*

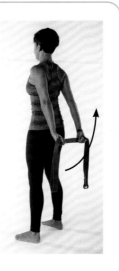

2. FULL BODY SIDE BEND

Stand with your feet hip-width apart. Sweep your arms up overhead and interlink your fingers. Now lean to the side aiming not to tip forwards or backwards. To go deeper, try clasping the top wrist and side bending further. *Hold for 20 seconds.*

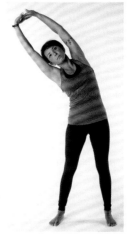

3. CHEST AND SHOULDER STRETCH WITH STRAP

Take your arms behind your back and interlink your hands. Lift your chest, draw your shoulders back and raise your hands. Do not lean forward. Lift your hands higher to go deeper. *Hold for 20 seconds.*

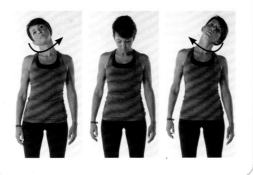

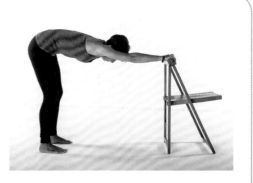

4. 90-DEGREE CHAIR STRETCH

Stand behind a chair and place your hands on the top of the chair back, shoulder-width apart. Walk backwards until you fold into a 90-degree position. To exit, walk forwards, bend your knees, draw the abdomen in and rise up to a standing position. *Hold for 20 seconds.*

5. ANCHORED QUAD STRETCH

Stand with your back to a chair. Lift your left leg up behind you and hook your toes onto the top of the chair (if the chair back is too high, try a lower surface such as a table). Bend your right leg a little and push your hips forward. Repeat on the other side. *Hold for 20 seconds.*

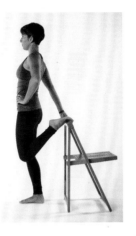

6. CHAIR BACK BEND

Hold onto the sides of the chair, lift your chest and squeeze your shoulder blades together. Gaze ahead or tuck the chin in. *Hold for 20 seconds.*

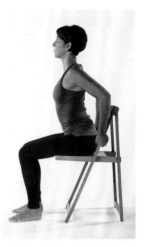

7. WIDE-LEGGED HALFWAY FORWARD BEND

Step the feet wide and turn your toes slightly inwards. Place your hands on your hips and tip your upper body forwards, stopping when your back begins to round. Remain here, or place your hands on the floor. *Hold for 30 seconds.*

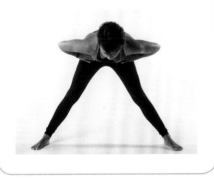

8. LYING PIGEON

Lie on your back and draw your right leg in towards your chest. Hold onto your right knee with your left hand and draw your leg across your body. Repeat on the other side. *Hold for 30 seconds.*

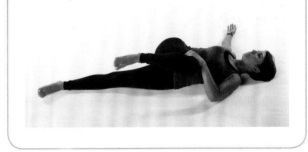

Total Body Flexibility: Intermediate Sequences

The Intermediate routines feature some advanced stretches attempted with the use of a cotton yoga strap, tie or dressing gown belt handy to bridge any gaps. There will be stretches you find easy while your body seems stubbornly resistant to others! So do substitute techniques from either the Gentle or Advanced sequences to create your own tailored routine.

Sequence 1

1. ARM WRAP STRETCH

Stand tall. Wrap your arms around your shoulders as if giving yourself a hug. Draw your shoulders away from your ears. *Hold for 20 seconds.*

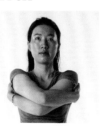

2. ADVANCED TRICEPS STRETCH (WITH STRAP)

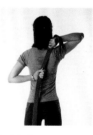

Remain standing. Lay a strap, belt or tie over your left shoulder. Reach up with your right arm and bend it so your hand drops behind your upper back. Take your left arm behind your back and slide it up the spine. Use the strap to bridge the gap between your hands. Repeat on the other side. *Hold for 20 seconds.*

3. KNEELING CALF STRETCH

Perform a Lunge by starting on all fours and stepping your right foot up between your hands. Shift your body weight back and roll your front foot onto the heel. Point your toes up. Repeat on the other side. *Hold for 20 seconds.*

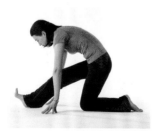

4. LOW LUNGE

On all fours, step your right foot up in between your hands and raise your upper body. Push your hips forward. Slowly lower into the lunge. Repeat on the other side. *Hold for 30 seconds.*

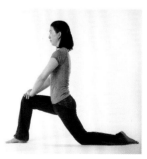

5. SPHINX

Lie down on your front, positioning your elbows directly under your shoulders with your forearms parallel. Draw your shoulder blades slightly closer together. *Hold for 20 seconds.*

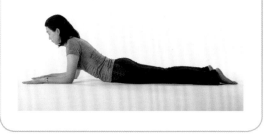

6. FIGURE FOUR

Lie on your back with your legs bent. Lift your right foot off the floor and turn your knee out. Rest your right ankle on top of your left thigh. Stay here or lift the feet off the floor and draw both legs in towards you. Hold behind the front thigh or clasp the front shin. Repeat on the other side. *Hold for 30 seconds.*

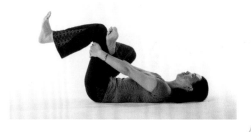

7. ADVANCED LYING TWIST 1

Lying on your back, loop a strap around your right foot. Hold onto both parts of the strap with your left hand and slowly draw your right leg across your body. Stretch your right arm out and turn your head to the right. Repeat on the other side. *Hold for 30 seconds.*

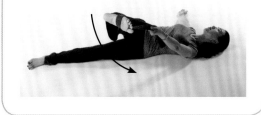

8. LYING HAMSTRING STRAP STRETCH

Lie on your back and loop a strap, belt or tie around the sole of the right foot. Bend the left leg and place your foot on the floor, especially if your hamstrings are tight. Straighten your right leg or keep it a little bent. Repeat on the other side. *Hold for 30 seconds.*

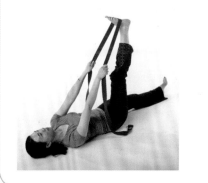

Sequence 2

1. ASSISTED SIDE NECK STRETCH

Lower your right ear to your right shoulder. Now raise your right arm up and place your right palm onto the left side of your head. Gently draw your head a little further over to the right. Repeat on the other side. *Hold for 10 seconds.*

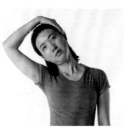

2. FULL BODY SIDE BEND

Stand with your feet hip-width apart. Sweep your arms up overhead and interlink your fingers. Now lean to the side aiming not to tip forwards or backwards. Clasp the top wrist and try bending further. *Hold for 20 seconds.*

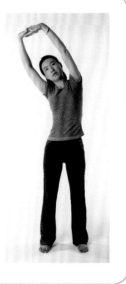

3. CHEST AND SHOULDER STRETCH WITH HANDS CLASPED

Take your arms behind your back and interlink your hands. Lift your chest, draw your shoulders back and raise your hands. Do not lean forward. Lift your hands higher to go deeper. *Hold for 20 seconds.*

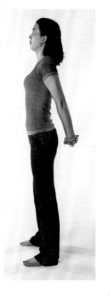

4. 90-DEGREE STRETCH

Stand with your feet hip-width apart. Tip your upper body forwards until you reach a 90-degree angle, or higher. Do not allow your back to curve. Place your hands on your thighs just above your knees. Fold lower if comfortable. *Hold for 20 seconds.*

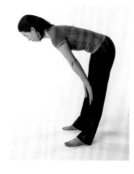

5. LYING QUAD STRETCH

Lower down onto your front. Bend your left leg and reach around for your foot. Press your hips into the floor and draw your leg closer to your buttocks. Repeat on the other side. *Hold for 20 seconds.*

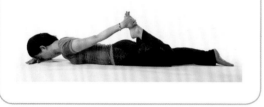

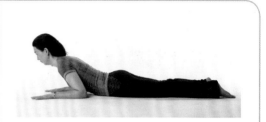

6. COBRA

Lie on your front with your hands under your shoulders. Press into your hands and slowly lift your upper body off the ground. Lower down and sit back on your heels. *Hold for 20 seconds.*

7. WIDE-LEGGED FORWARD BEND

Step your feet wide and turn your toes slightly inwards. Place your hands on your hips and tip your upper body forwards, stopping when your back begins to round. Remain here, or place your hands on the floor. *Hold for 30 seconds.*

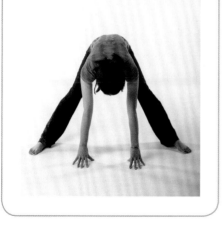

8. PIGEON

Begin on all fours. Slide your right knee up behind your right wrist. Wiggle your right foot a little over to the left. Straighten your back leg. Lower yourself slowly either onto your forearms or stack one hand on top of the other and rest your forehead on your hands. Repeat on the other side. *Hold for 30 seconds.*

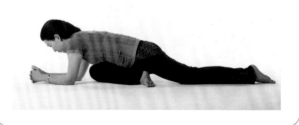

Total Body Flexibility: Advanced Sequences

These final advanced sequences are designed for the naturally supple, or as aspirational routines for those wishing to progress with regular stretching to become more flexible. However, as with all stretching, only move to the point of tension, never discomfort or pain. Having a good degree of flexibility does not mean you can launch into this sequence with cold muscles, so please raise your body temperature with some simple movements, such as marching on the spot and rolling your shoulders in circles.

Sequence 1

1. ADVANCED ARM WRAP

Stand tall. Wrap your right arm over your left to cross your arms. Now bring your palms closer or touching. Draw your shoulders away from your ears. Unravel and repeat, crossing your left arm over the right. *Hold for 20 seconds.*

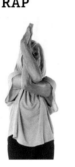

2. ADVANCED TRICEPS STRETCH

Remain standing. Reach up with your right arm and bend it so your hand drops behind your upper back. Take your left arm behind your back and slide your hand up your spine towards the middle of your shoulder blades. Clasp your hands together or use a strap to bridge the gap. Repeat on the other side. *Hold for 20 seconds.*

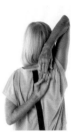

3. DOWNWARD FACING DOG

Start on all fours. Spread your fingers wide. Lift your hips up to make a triangle shape with your body. Press both heels down towards the floor. *Hold for 30 seconds.*

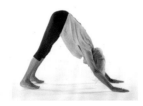

4. LOW LUNGE WITH QUAD STRETCH

Start on all fours. Perform the low lunge by stepping your left foot up between your hands. Lean a little to the left, nd bend your right leg. Reach around to hold your right foot. Shift your weight back to the centre and lift your upper body. Repeat on the other side. *Hold for 20 seconds.*

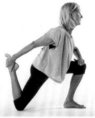

5. STRIKING COBRA

Lie on your front with your hand just under your shoulders. Press into your hands and slowly raise your upper body off the ground. *Hold for 10 seconds.* Lower yourself down and sit back on your heels.

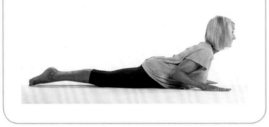

6. LYING LEG KNOT

Lie on your back with your legs bent. Cross your right leg over your left at thigh level and hug both legs in towards you. Hold just below your top knee or clasp both feet. Switch legs by crossing the left leg on top. *Hold for 20 seconds.*

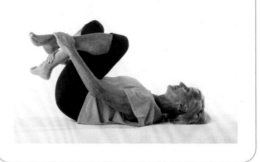

7. ADVANCED LYING TWIST 2

Bend both legs and place your feet on the floor. Stretch your arms out shoulder-height, palms facing upwards. Lower both legs down to the floor on the right side and straighten them. Either hold onto your toes with your right hand or loop a strap around the soles of your feet and hold the strap. *Hold for 30 seconds.*

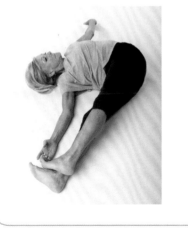

8. ADVANCED LYING HAMSTRING STRETCH

Lie on your back. Lift your left leg up towards the ceiling. Straighten your right leg and rest it on the floor. Hold behind your thigh and draw your leg closer towards you. You may be able to walk your hands higher up to your foot or grasp your toes with your left hand. *Hold for 30 seconds.*

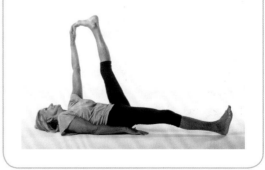

Sequence 2

1. CLASPED HANDS NECK STRETCH

Take your hands behind your back. Interlink them and slide them around the right side of your waist. Tip your head over to the right. Repeat on the other side. *Hold for 10 seconds.*

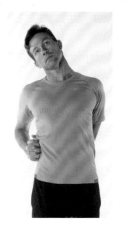

2. TRIANGLE

Step your feet wide, turn your right foot out 90-degrees and your left foot slightly inwards. Raise your arms up to shoulder height. Tip your upper body to the right. Lightly rest your right hand on your leg. Either reach your left arm up or reach it over by your left ear to perform the more advanced version. Repeat on the other side. *Hold for 30 seconds.*

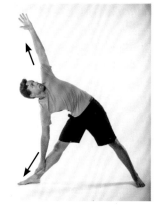

3. ADVANCED CHEST AND SHOULDER STRETCH

Take your arms behind your back and interlink your hands. Bend your knees, tip forwards from the hips, drop your head and lift your hands off the lower back. Remain here for 20-30 seconds letting the weight of the arms drop forwards. To exit, drop your hands to the lower back, bend your knees deeply and rise up to a standing position with a flat back. *Hold for 20 seconds.*

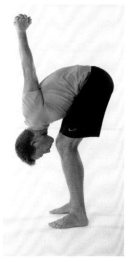

4. FULL FORWARD BEND

Stand with your feet hip-width apart and a slight bend in your knees. Fold forward and place either your fingertips or palms on the floor either side of your feet. Exit carefully by bending your knees deeper, pulling in your abdomen and rising up to a standing position with a straight back. *Hold for 30 seconds.*

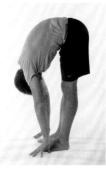

5. DYNAMIC QUAD STRETCH

Stand tall with your feet hip-width apart. Slowly bend your left leg and reach around to hold your left foot with your left hand. Hold onto a chair for balance if required. Push your hips forward. Bend your right leg and draw your left leg back further. Now start to move your leg by alternately pointing your knee forward and drawing your knee back. Repeat on the other side. *Repeat x 4.*

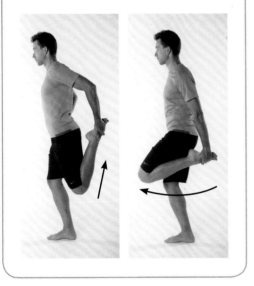

6. SNAKE

Lie on your front with your hands interlocked behind your back. Lift your upper body and legs a little off the floor. Tuck your chin in so you are looking down, not forwards. *Hold for 10 seconds.*

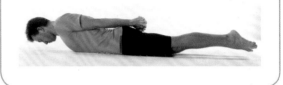

7. WIDE-LEGGED SEATED STRETCH

Sit tall with your legs stretched out wide and toes pointing upward. Keeping a straight spine, begin to walk your hands forwards until you feel your back and inner thigh muscles stretching. *Hold for 30 seconds.*

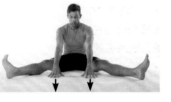

8. PIGEON

Begin on all fours. Slide your right knee up behind your right wrist. Wiggle your right foot a little over to the left. Straighten your back leg. Stack one hand on top of the other and rest your forehead on your hands. *Hold for 30 seconds.*

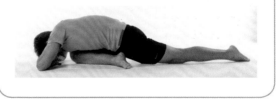

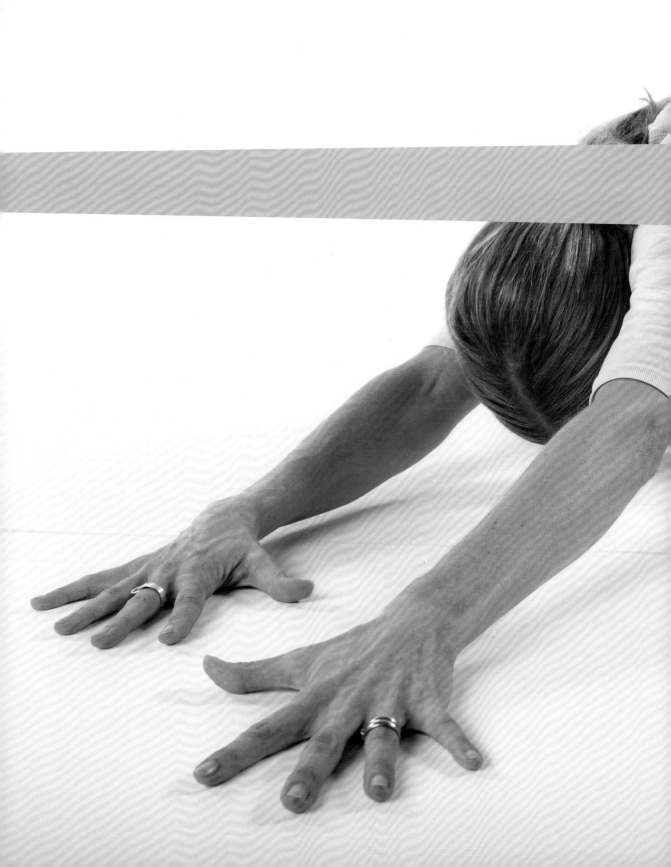

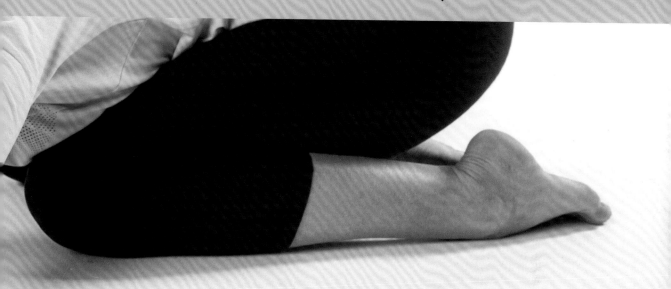

Stretches by Sport

The Warm-Up

The Benefits of Warming Up

To avoid injury

The purpose of the warm-up is to increase heart rate, raise the core body temperature and get the blood flowing through dynamic, limbering movements. The muscles are warmed and prepared for sport by working through various ranges of motion. This improves tissue elasticity and reduces the risk of muscle or tendon injury. By the time the athlete sidesteps into a deep lunge in tennis or twists his body to fire a soccer ball into the net, his muscles are pliant and ready.

> **WARNING: SAVE THE DEEP, STATIC STRETCHING**
>
> Holding deep, static stretches prior to a workout is now thought to actually impede, rather than improve performance. Studies have shown that it can decrease speed, strength and power. This particularly includes any sport that requires explosive bursts of power and strength such as sprinting or long jump as well as shorter swims and weightlifting. This is why we save long-held stretching for the post-sport cool down.

To enter the zone

The warm-up has a psychological as well as physiological purpose as it shifts the athlete's focus onto the game, match, run or ride ahead. The familiar and repetitive sequence of a warm-up can also be comforting and requires concentration, leaving those athletes who suffer with nerves no time to become anxious or distracted.

To practise movement patterns

Warm-ups that particularly focus on mimicking the movement patterns of the athlete's sport will allow them to practise skills such as coordination, balance, speed and agility as well as improving range of motion in the muscle groups used for that sport. By the time the athlete walks onto the court, track or pitch, the muscles are primed and movement patterns ingrained in her mind.

To bond as a team

For team sports, the warm-up is a chance to cement bonds especially if warm-ups are done with partners. Performing warm-up techniques with a partner also ensures that a good pace or momentum is maintained. Here are just a handful of examples of partner warm-up techniques, some of which are adapted from stretches in the sport-specific sections of this chapter (for static, or long-held, stretches to try with a partner *after* exercise see *Post-Exercise Partner Cool Downs* on page 163).

PRE-EXERCISE PARTNER WARM-UPS

Repeat each partner warm-up x 4-6

1. LEG SWING

Stand to the right side of your partner and place your hand on their shoulder. Your partner will place their hand on your shoulder. Both of you swing your outer legs back and forth. Simply both turn 180 degrees to face the other direction to repeat the swinging action with the other leg.

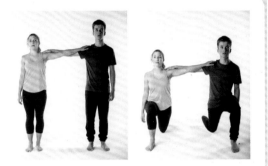

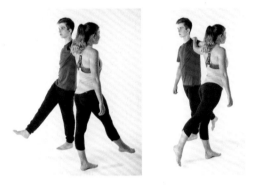

3. LUNGES

Take a step forwards with one leg so that when you bend your front leg to a 90-degree angle, the ankle is directly over your front knee. Simultaneously drop your back knee down so that it hovers above the floor.

4. SQUAT

Face your partner with your feet wide and toes slightly turned out. Cross your arms at the wrists and hold hands. Now lower into a squat simultaneously and rise up together. Take care to maintain a straight spine and lower just far enough so that you can still see your toes.

2. SIDE LEG SWING

This is similar to the Leg Swing but your legs move laterally, out to the side and across the body.

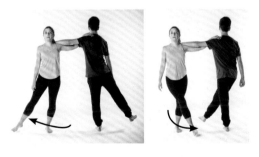

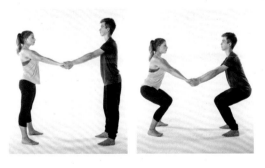

The All Sport Warm-Up Sequence

How to use the sequence

This whole body warm-up sequence is applicable for all sports. The dynamic or moving stretches will raise the heart rate and get the blood flowing to general muscle groups, beginning with the feet and ankles and working gradually upwards to the neck and shoulders.

You can use the sequence in any of the three following ways:

1 Run through the entire sequence, repeating each technique four times. This should take a maximum of ten minutes.

2 Select the warm-ups that best mimic the movement patterns you make in your sport.

Or for a tailor-made, sport-specific warm-up, locate your sport in *Stretches by Sport* and perform the six warm-up techniques suggested.

Repeat each warm up x 4.

1. ANKLE ROLL

Place your hands on your hips. Stand on your left leg and lift your right foot off the floor. Rotate your foot slowly. Repeat on the other side.

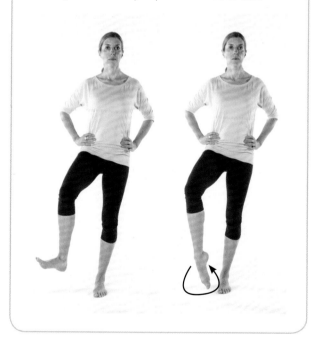

2. HEEL AND TOE ROCKING

Rock your weight back into the heels and lift your toes off the floor. Rock your weight forwards onto the balls of your feet and lift your heels off the floor.

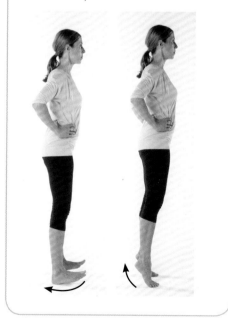

3. KNEE CIRCLE

Stand with your feet together and bend your legs. Place your hands on your knees. Make circles with your knees.

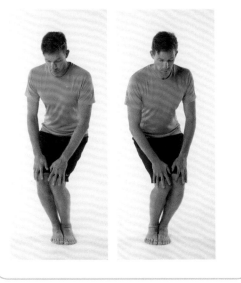

4. HIP CIRCLE

Place your hands on your hips and make large, smooth circles with your hips keeping a slight bend in your knees.

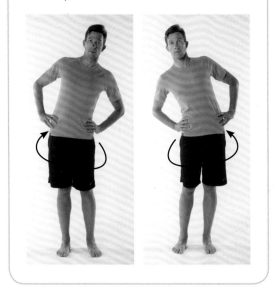

5. LEG SWING

Stand on your left leg and slowly swing your right leg back and forth. Let your arms swing freely in opposition to mimic walking or running. Switch legs.

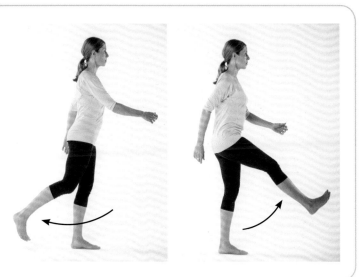

6. SIDE LEG SWING

Stand on your left leg and slowly swing your right leg across your body back and forth. Rest your right hand on a wall for support if required. Switch legs.

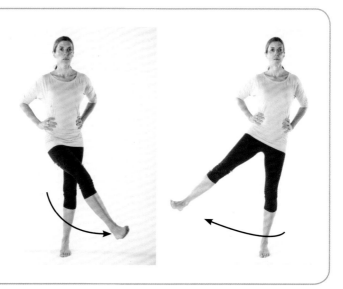

7. BACK KICKS

Stand on your left leg. Bend your right leg as if trying to kick your buttocks. Switch from leg to leg.

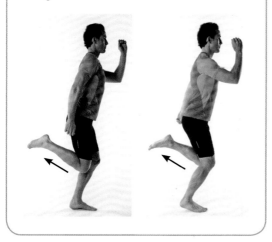

8. MARCHING

Perform a marching action by walking on the spot, lifting your knees high. Position your arms in a right angle shape and swing them back and forth.

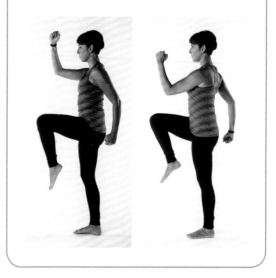

9. HEEL TAP

Stand on your right leg. Lift your left leg up, bend it and turn your knee out. Tap your left heel with your right hand. Switch from leg to leg.

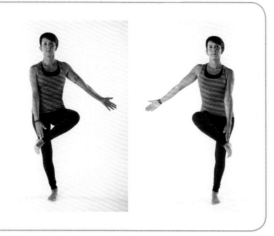

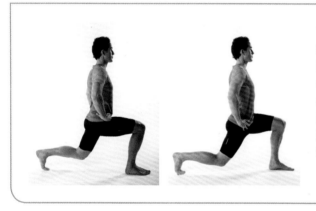

10. LUNGE

Place your hands on your hips. Take a large step forwards with your right leg and bend your knee to a 90-degree angle, ensuring your ankle is over your knee. Simultaneously drop your back knee down so that it hovers above the floor. Step back to standing.

11. LUNGE WITH TWIST

Fold your arms and hold on to your elbows. As you step forwards with your right foot, rotate your upper body to the right. Rotate to face forwards and step back to standing. Repeat on the other side.

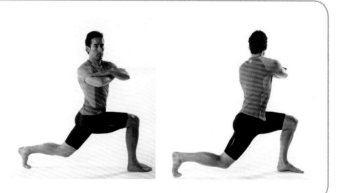

12. SUMO SQUATS

Place your hands on your hips. Step your feet wide with your toes slightly turned outwards. Bend both legs and lower into a squat checking that your knees are aligned with your second toes and your toes are just visible in the squat. Rise back up to standing.

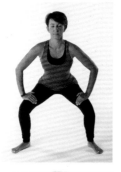

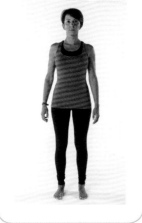

13. SPEED SKATER

Step your feet wider with your toes slightly turned outwards. Lower into a side lunge by bending your right leg and straightening your left. Sweep your left arm across your chest and drop your left elbow down. Let your upper body twist a little. Lunge from side to side.

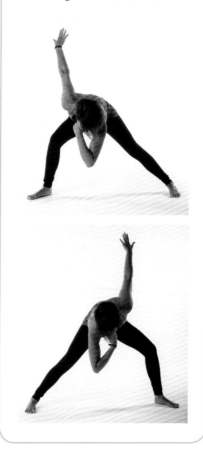

14. DYNAMIC SIDE BENDING

Stand with your feet hip-width apart. Sweep your left arm up and tip over to the right, trying not to lean forwards or backwards. Return to the centre. Sweep the right arm up and tip to the left.

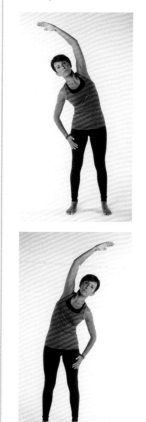

15. STANDING TWIST

Bend your knees a little and relax your arms by your sides. Twist your upper body to the right and let the arms swing around. Return to the centre and twist to the left.

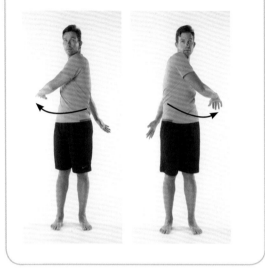

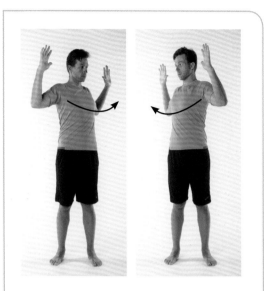

16. MID-BACK WARM-UP

Move your arms into a 90-degree position. Keep your hips and legs still and twist your upper body slowly and gently from side to side.

17. SWIMMING ARMS 1

Drop your fingertips onto your shoulders and 'swim' your arms by making alternate circles with your elbows. Roll your shoulders first forwards, then in a backwards motion.

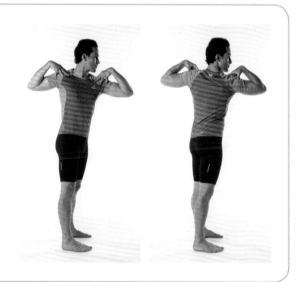

18. SWIMMING ARMS 2

'Swim' your arms mimicking a front crawl movement. Allow your upper body to rotate as you reach forwards with alternate arms. Reverse the exercise by copying the backstroke movement.

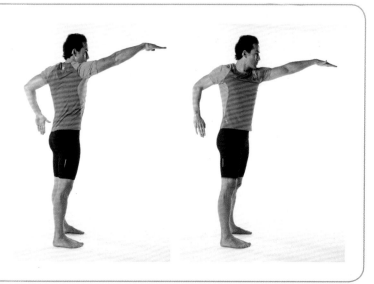

19. WRIST AND HAND WARMER

Interlace your fingers, palms down and chest-height. Pull your hands slightly apart as if your fingers were stuck together until you can feel some traction. Then, alternately flex and extend (bend and draw back) your wrists.

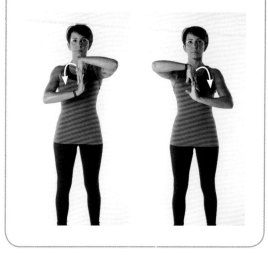

20. HEAD ROLL

Make a continuous semi-circle movement with your head by first tipping your head to the right side by dropping your ear to your shoulder, looking down at your feet, then rolling your head around to the left shoulder. Move in slow motion. Don't tip your head back. Repeat in the other direction.

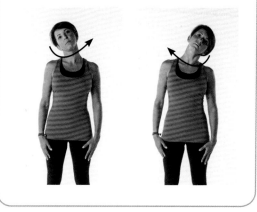

Speed It Up:
The Dynamic Warm-Up

Some of the warm-up stretches in the All Sport Warm-Up Sequence can be speeded up and made more energetic to forge a more energetic routine that will quickly get the heart pumping and boost your body temperature. This is particularly useful in cold weather and great for sports that require running, sprinting or rapid changes of direction such as rugby, football, basketball or hockey.

The dynamic touch comes from traversing forward or sideways, by running, hopping or jumping. For example, rather than warming up the quads by staying on the spot and drawing each heel to buttock (see step 7: Back Kicks), the athlete can hop lightly from foot to foot.

These dynamic techniques often also mimic movements and muscle recruitment patterns used in the athlete's sport. For example, the Traversing Lunge and Back Kick Walking break down the running stride making these moving techniques very useful for runners. They also improve not just flexibility training, but often also strength, balance and coordination.

Be warned though: dynamic stretching carries an increased risk of injury and can be tough on the joints. Play it safe by performing light, aerobic activity such as jogging for five minutes and only progress to hopping or jumping movements if you are strong and injury-free.

Here are some examples of dynamic warm-ups:

1. BACK KICK WALKING

Walk forwards, kicking your back heel up towards your buttocks. Or, for a more dynamic version, perform it hopping from leg to leg.

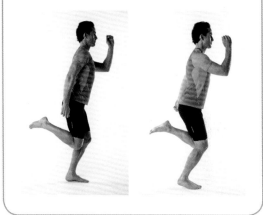

2. BALANCED BACK KICK WALKING

Walk forwards, kicking your back heel up towards your buttocks. Pause as your right heel is lifted and reach around to draw your heel further in with the right hand. Simultaneously rise onto the ball of your left foot. Avoid leaning forwards by maintaining an upright spine. Lower and repeat on the other side.

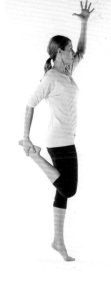

3. TOY SOLDIER

Stand on your left leg and swing your right leg through. Repeat, moving forwards like a toy soldier with straight legs. Start with low legs, but lift each leg higher after a few steps.

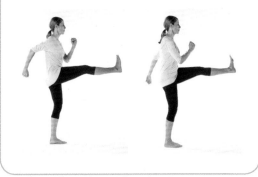

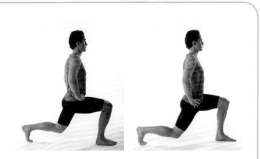

4. TRAVERSING LUNGE

Take a large step forwards with your right leg and drop your left knee downwards so that it hovers above the floor. Step up with your left leg. Continue to travel forwards alternating legs.

5. TRAVERSING LUNGE WITH TWIST

Fold your arms across your chest. Take a large step forwards with your right leg into the lunge and twist your upper body to the right. Step up with the left leg. Continue to travel forwards alternating legs.

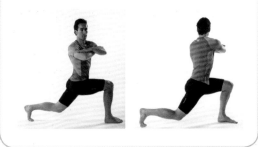

6. TRAVERSING SUMO SQUATS

Do wide Sumo-style side lunges by taking a step out to the side, bending both knees to drop into the squat. Position your toes slightly turned outwards. You should be able to still see your toes as you sit into the squat. Traverse to the right side, then traverse to the left.

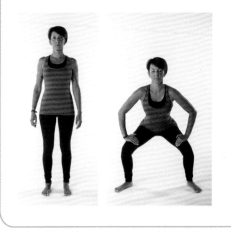

The Cool Down

The Benefits of the Cool Down

To increase power

Regular post-sport static stretching (held for 20, 30 or 60 seconds) can also boost performance by allowing the athlete to exert maximum force through a wider range of motion. Not all sports, of course, require a good range of motion, but a tennis forehand, golf swing or throwing a javelin are just three actions that use flexibility to release power. Picture how a golfer's hips, torso and shoulders coil back to unleash the swing.

Please note: static stretching *prior* to exercise can have the opposite effect of decreasing power so save deep muscle lengthening until after the game, match, run or ride.

To recover faster

Athletes who regularly stretch often find that it increases exercise tolerance. What this means is that by reducing post-exercise aches or pains they are able to run, cycle or ski sooner and for longer. Stretching can reduce Delayed Onset Muscle Soreness (DOMS) or the stiffness that occurs between 24-48 hours after exercise. Personally, I find this works best if I stretch once immediately after exercise when the muscles are still warm and then again for 20 minutes just before bedtime. Of course, this reduction in

> ### STRETCH *AND* STRENGTHEN FOR INJURY PREVENTION
>
> It is important to emphasise here that, although this is a stretching book, sometimes injuries are due to a combination of 'tight' muscles and weak muscles, so stretching and strengthening should go hand in hand. Your coach or physiotherapist will be able to create a conditioning plan that addresses both elements of injury prevention.

soreness will depend a lot on the intensity and duration of exercise. Remember: only perform light stretches if the muscles are very sore.

To avoid injury

As with the warm-up, stretching is thought to help avoid injury, though this still remains anecdotal rather than based on firm scientific evidence. Some research suggests that it is the warm-up rather than the post-sport stretch that better prevents injury. It does seem to be common sense that increasing an athlete's range of movement will increase the distance she can extend or flex her limbs before damage occurs to muscles and tendons. For example, footballer's hamstrings can more easily respond to him kicking a ball without injury if they are supple and pliant. Whether this is due to the pre-match warm-up, the post-match cool-down stretch, or a combination of both, is still under discussion in the sports science community.

To gain performance-enhancing flexibility

Most athletes want to stretch purely to avoid injury and gain an appropriate range of motion for their sport. Some sports, however, demand a high level of flexibility for improved performance. At one end of this scale are sports such as kickboxing or Taekwondo, but professional swimmers also have amazingly supple upper bodies. This allows them to reduce turbulence and slide smoothly and efficiently through the water. If you are interested in becoming noticeably more flexible in order to aid performance, see *How to Become a Super Supple Athlete* box on the right.

To do the sport you love for longer

This is the benefit that I find most athletes can relate to – even those highly resistant to the idea of stretching. Regular flexibility work creates longevity. In other words, it allows you to cycle, kayak or play tennis for longer. By longer I mean on that particular morning or day, but it can also extend the number of years you can train or compete. There are numerous examples of professional sportspeople who have lengthened their careers through diligent and regular stretching, such as Manchester United's soccer star Ryan Giggs who was still playing at the age of 40. Giggs credited the longevity of his career largely to his yoga practice and became a key proponent of yoga for soccer players.

HOW TO BECOME A SUPER SUPPLE ATHLETE

Most sportspeople simply stretch to avoid injury or aching muscles and do the minimum required. If, however, your sport demands a high level of flexibility, you'll need to do more than the post-exercise routines provided later in this chapter. First the bad news: some of us are born bendy as the composition of elastin and collagen of our connective tissue is largely determined at birth. The good news is that, with dedication, you will see gains although over a matter of weeks rather than days. The secret to seeing gains is little and often. Studies have shown that range of motion can be increased by a single 15-30 second stretch for each muscle group, but this should be done daily or even twice daily. Choose a simple stretch such as the Leg-Up Hamstring Stretch (page 81) that can be done easily, even in the office. Perform the stretch three times. Dedication will reap rewards.

POST-EXERCISE PARTNER COOL DOWNS

In the warm-up section, we looked at assisted or partner warm-ups to encourage team bonding and provide stability where balance is required. Team members can also work together in post-play static stretching. Here are four examples of techniques done with a partner.

Warning: if you are doing the stretching move slowly and gently. If you are being stretched ask your partner to stop at the 'edge' of the stretch so you have room to go deeper if required. Breathe deeply throughout. Communicate regularly with your partner. If you are assisting with the stretch, ask your partner for continual feedback and watch their expressions for any sign of discomfort. *Hold each stretch for 30 seconds.*

1. ANTERIOR SHOULDER STRETCH

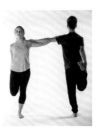

Stand tall with your partner behind you. Raise both arms up horizontally. Allow your partner to hold your hands or wrists and gently draw your arms backwards while you maintain a straight spine. Stop when you feel the point of tension.

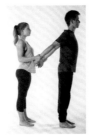

2. STANDING QUAD STRETCH

Stand to the right of your partner and place your hands on each other's shoulders. Stand tall. Now both bend your outside legs, reach back with your right hands and gently draw your heels in towards your hips. Maintain a straight spine and push your hips forwards.

3. PARTNER BUTTERFLY

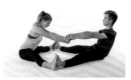

Sit on the ground facing your partner. Take your legs wide and place the soles of your feet together. Hold hands and sit tall. Either remain here or gently draw your partner a little further forward by leaning back. *Hold for 30-60 seconds and then ask your partner to lean back.*

4. SEATED PECTORAL STRETCH

Sit on the ground. Sit tall and clasp your hands behind your head. Relax your shoulders. Ask your partner to stand behind you, hold your elbows and gently draw your arms back.

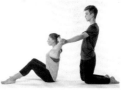

5. LYING HAMSTRING STRETCH

Lie on the ground with the legs bent and feet on the floor. Raise your left leg up. Your partner will either stand or kneel beside your leg and gently push it towards you. If you have good hamstring flexibility, this stretch can be performed with the right leg extended along the floor, otherwise keep the right leg bent.

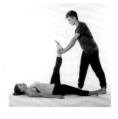

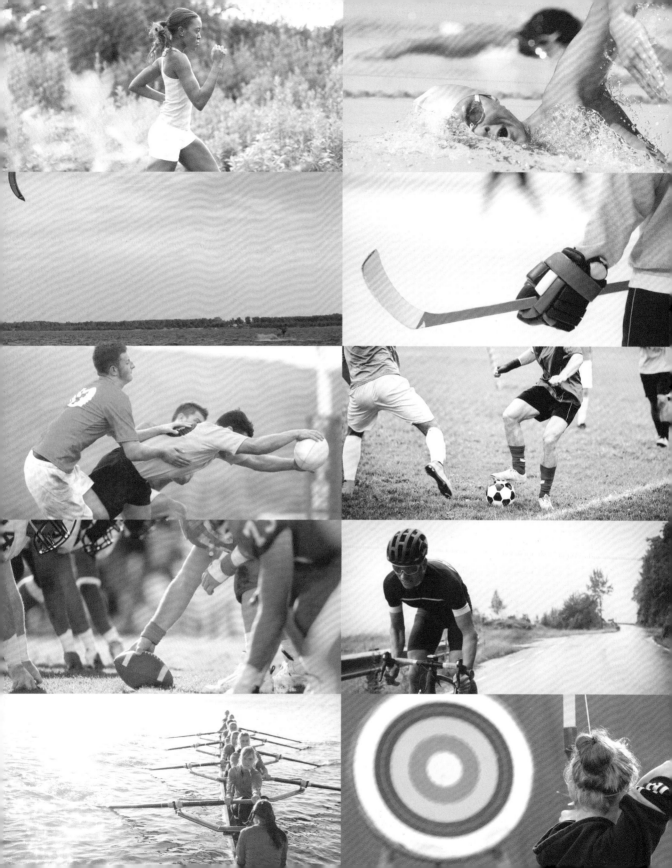

The following section breaks down stretching by sport. Each of the 20 sport sections features six warm-ups and 10 post-exercise still or static stretches. In addition, there is an extra advanced 'Going Deeper' stretch to try as flexibility improves or for the naturally more supple athlete. The sequences are designed to flow in a logical order with most beginning in the standing position and moving down to the floor.

Perform a brisk walk or light jog for 5-10 minutes before commencing the warm-up. Repeat each warm-up 4-6 times and hold each post-sport stretch for 30 seconds (or longer if the muscles feel very tight).

American Football

The following pre- and post-game stretch sequence focuses on priming and stretching the muscles of the hips to ensure players can make multi-directional moves with agility without injury and are able to comfortably perform a low squat. The routine also targets the running/sprinting muscles and the shoulder and torso muscles involved in twisting and throwing the ball.

6 Warm-Ups for American Football

Repeat each stretch x 4

1. SWIMMING ARMS 2

Stand tall and 'swim' your arms, mimicking a front crawl movement. Allow your upper body to rotate as you reach forwards with alternate arms. Reverse the exercise by copying the backstroke movement.

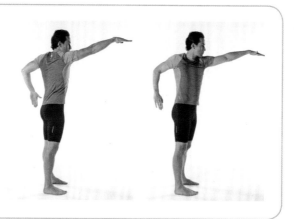

2. HEEL TAP

Stand on your right leg. Lift your left leg up, bend it and turn your knee out. Tap your left heel with your right hand. Switch from leg to leg.

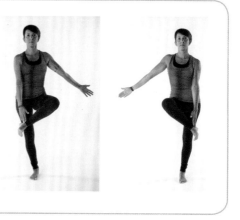

3. TOY SOLDIER

Stand on your right leg and swing your left leg through. Repeat, moving forwards like a toy soldier with straight legs. Start with low legs, but lift each leg higher after a few steps.

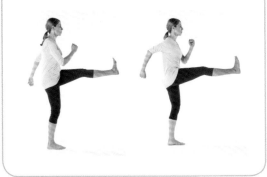

4. BALANCED BACK KICK WALKING

Walk forwards and kick your back heel up towards your buttocks. Reach around and hold your foot to draw your heel in. As you do this, rise onto the ball of the foot. Avoid leaning forwards by ensuring your upper body remains upright.

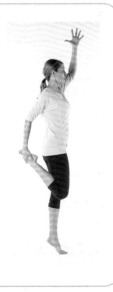

5. THE WALKING LUNGE WITH TWIST

Fold your arms across your chest. Take a large step forwards with your right leg into the lunge and twist your upper body to the right. Step up with your left leg. Continue to travel forwards alternating legs.

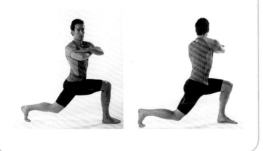

6. TRAVERSING SUMO SQUATS

Do wide Sumo-style side lunges by taking a step out to the side, bending both knees to drop into the squat. Position your toes slightly turned outwards. You should be able to still see your toes as you sit into the squat. Traverse to the right side, then traverse to the left.

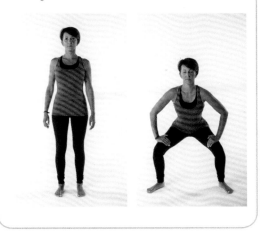

10 Post-American Football Stretches

Hold each stretch for 20–30 seconds

1. TRICEPS STRETCH

Stand with your feet hip-width apart. Reach up with your right arm and bend it so your hand drops behind your upper back. Use your left hand to gently draw your right elbow back. Repeat on the other side.

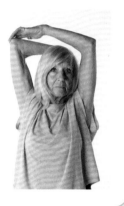

2. OVERHEAD STRAP STRETCH

Stand with your feet hip-width apart. Raise your strap, tie or belt overhead with your hands wide. Bend your arms until they form a 90-degree angle and draw your elbows back.

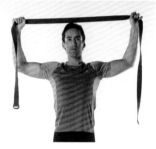

3. WIDE-LEGGED FORWARD BEND

Step your feet wide and turn your toes slightly inwards. Place your hands on your hips and tip your upper body forwards, stopping when your back begins to round. Remain here, or place your hands on the floor.

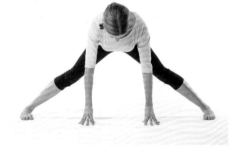

4. LOW LUNGE

Lower yourself down to all fours. Step your right foot up in between your hands and raise your upper body. Push your hips forward. Slowly lower yourself into the lunge. Repeat on the other side.

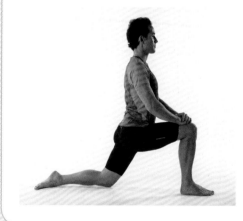

5. LOW LUNGE WITH SIDE BEND

Remain in the low lunge. Reach high with your left arm and lean your upper body over to the right. Keep pushing your hips forwards. Repeat on the other side.

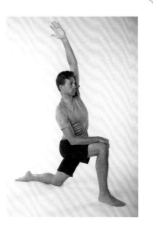

6. BUTTERFLY

Sit either on the floor, or the edge of a cushion if you find it hard to straighten your spine. Bring the soles of your feet together. Clasp your hands around your feet or ankles and sit tall.

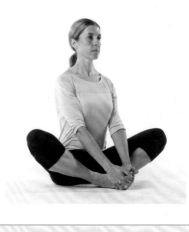

7. ALL FOURS MID-BACK TWIST

Move to all fours, but with your knees wide apart. Ensure your hands are directly under your shoulders.

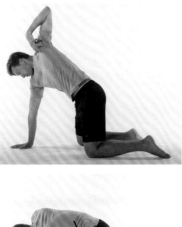

Place your left hand on your left shoulder. Stay looking down. As you inhale, point your left elbow up to the ceiling. As you exhale, point your left elbow under your right armpit. Repeat x 4 and then repeat on the other side.

8. KNEELING BACK STRETCH

Lower down to sit on the heels. Straighten your arms and reach your hands out in front of you. Spread your fingers and press down. Now draw your hips away in the opposite direction.

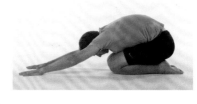

9. LYING QUAD STRETCH

Lower down onto your front. Bend your right leg and reach around for your foot. Press your pelvis into the floor to avoid arching your back and draw the leg closer to your buttocks. Repeat on the other side.

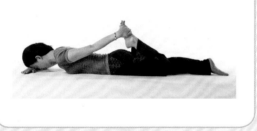

10. FIGURE FOUR SITTING

Sit on the floor with your legs bent. Lift your right foot off the floor and turn your knee out. Rest your right ankle on top of your left thigh. Stay here or lift the feet off the floor and draw both legs in towards you. Hold behind your front thigh or clasp your front shin. Repeat on the other side.

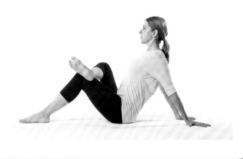

GOING DEEPER: LIZARD

Lizard is basically a very low lunge with a deep groin stretch to release muscles worked in the squat position, running and sprinting. Lizard also stretches the hip flexor in the back leg. You may need to pad the back knee with a block or cushion. It is also useful to have foam yoga or Pilates blocks or a pile of books handy to rest your forearms on.

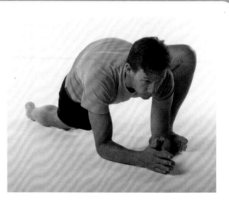

From all fours, step your left foot up to the outside of your left hand. Let your hips sink down. Either remain with straight arms or slowly lower down onto your forearms. A block or book under each forearm will raise the floor level if this proves difficult. Uncurl your back toes so the front of your foot rests on the floor. You can roll onto the edge of your left foot and drop your left knee out to the side to create more space to drop lower into the lunge.

Archery and Shooting

The 'mental' sports such as archery, pistol or rifle shooting may be the least energetic category of sport, but holding the body stock still while you take aim is demanding, particularly on the muscles of the neck, shoulders and upper back. Stretching can also release tension in the lower back from prolonged standing and help prevent muscular imbalances from occurring from these asymmetrical or one-sided sports.

6 Warm-Ups for Archery and Shooting

Repeat each stretch x 4

1. STANDING TWIST

Bend your knees and relax your arms by your sides. Twist your upper body to the right and let your arms swing around. Return to the centre and twist to the left.

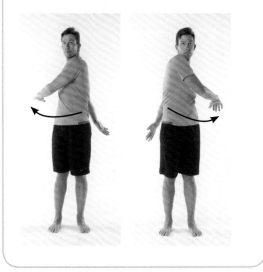

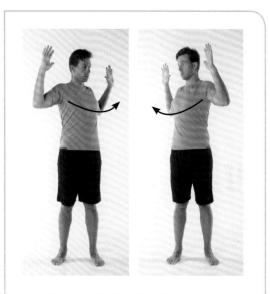

2. MID-BACK WARM UP

Move your arms into a 90-degree position. Keep your hips and legs still and twist your upper body slowly and gently from side to side.

3. DYNAMIC SIDE BENDING

Stand with your feet hip-width apart. Sweep your left arm up and tip over to the right, trying not to lean forwards or backwards. Return to the centre. Sweep the right arm up and tip to the left.

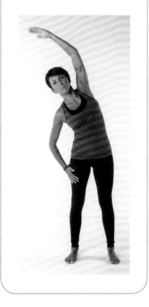

4. SWIMMING ARMS 1

Drop your fingertips onto your shoulders and 'swim' your arms by making alternate circles with your elbows. Roll your shoulders first forwards, then in a backwards motion.

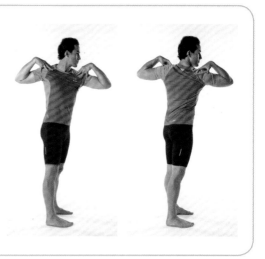

5. SQUEEZE AND SPREAD

Squeeze your hands into fists tucking the thumb in and hold for five seconds. Now spread your hands wide and hold for five seconds.

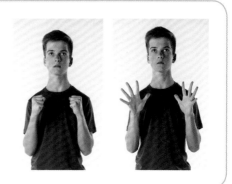

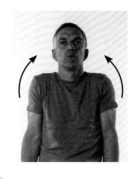

6. SHOULDER SHRUG

Lift your shoulders up towards your ears. Hold for a second. Now let them drop down.

10 Post-Archery and Shooting Stretches

Hold each stretch for 20–30 seconds

1. ASSISTED NECK EXTENSOR STRETCH

Interlink your hands behind your head. Drop your head down. Do not push your head further, but just let your elbows drop forwards so the weight of your arms increases the stretch.

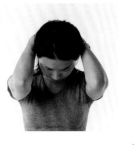

2. LATERAL NECK STRETCH

Stand tall with your arms by your sides. Look forwards. Slowly lower your right ear to your right shoulder. To go deeper, press your left shoulder downwards. Repeat on the other side.

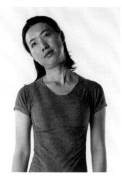

3. ROTATING NECK STRETCH

Stand tall. Keep your shoulders facing front. Slowly rotate your head to the right and then to left.

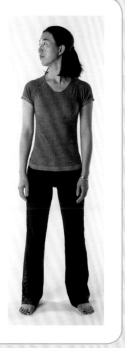

4. WRIST EXTENSOR STRETCH

Hold your right arm out straight. Grasp your right fingers and draw them back towards your palm. Repeat on the other side.

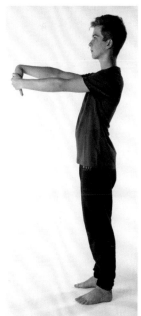

5. WRIST FLEXOR STRETCH

Hold your right arm out straight. Lift your fingers and draw them back towards your body. Repeat on the other side.

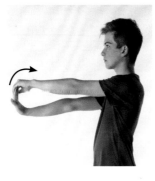

6. TRICEPS STRETCH

Stand with your feet hip-width apart. Reach up with your right arm and bend it so your hand drops behind your upper back. Use your left hand to gently draw your right elbow back. Repeat on the other side.

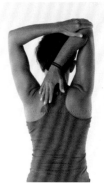

7. POSTERIOR SHOULDER STRETCH

Stand with your right arm straight and at chest height. Place your left hand behind your right elbow and draw your arm across your body. Do not rotate the torso. Repeat on the other side.

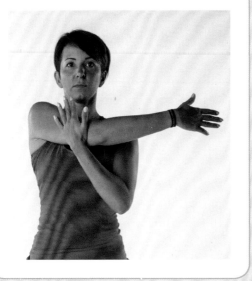

8. STANDING BACK BEND

Stand with your feet hip-width apart. Place your hands on your lower back, fingers pointing downwards. Lean back. Draw your elbows together. Lift your chin a little, but don't drop your head back.

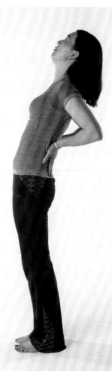

9. 90-DEGREE CHAIR STRETCH

Place your hands on the back of a chair shoulder-width apart or wider. Walk your feet back until your body tips into a 90-degree shape. Drop your head in line with your torso and pull your abdomen in so you are not dipping in the lower back.

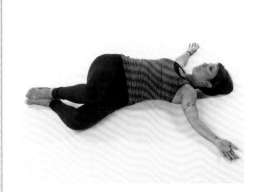

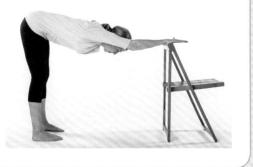

10. BASIC LYING TWIST

Bend both legs and place your feet on the floor. Stretch your arms out at shoulder height, palms facing upwards. Lower both legs down to the floor on the left side and relax them. Repeat on the other side.

GOING DEEPER: ADVANCED ARM WRAP

This is a deeper version of the Posterior Shoulder Stretch (stretch number 7). It may not be feasible if you have a wide chest or well developed arm/shoulder muscles.

Stand tall. Wrap your right arm over your left to cross your arms. Now bring your forearms closer to your face. Connect your palms if possible. Relax your shoulders away from your ears and tuck your chin in. Experiment with the following variations:

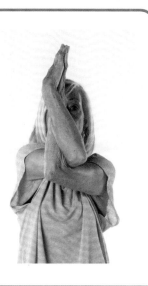

- Draw your arms downwards
- Lift your arms upwards
- Move your arms to the left
- Move your arms to the right

Unravel and repeat the stretch, crossing the left arm over the right.

Baseball and Softball

Baseball and softball players need superior flexibility in the shoulders. Stiffness in this area, through age or overuse, can start to negatively affect the power and speed of throwing and leave players susceptible to injuries such as tendonitis. Both games also require bursts of sprinting, torso rotation and low squatting, so warm-up and cool down stretches for the relevant muscle groups are included in the routine below.

6 Warm-Ups for Baseball and Softball

Repeat each stretch x 4

1. SWIMMING ARMS 1

Drop your fingertips onto your shoulders and 'swim' your arms by making alternate circles with your elbows. Roll your shoulders first forwards, then in a backwards motion.

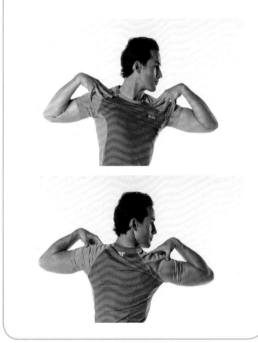

2. SWIMMING ARMS 2

Drop your fingertips onto your shoulders and 'swim' your arms by making alternate circles with your elbows. Roll your shoulders first forwards, then in a backwards motion.

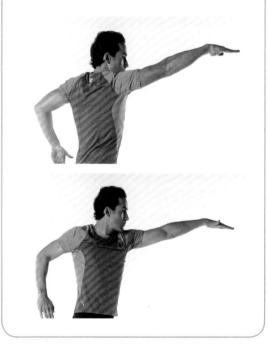

3. WRIST AND HAND WARMER

Interlace your fingers, palms down at chest-height. Pull your hands slightly apart as if your fingers were stuck together until you can feel some traction. Then, alternately flex and extend (bend and draw back) your wrists.

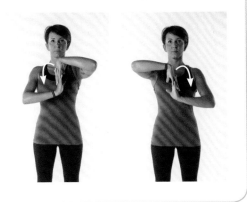

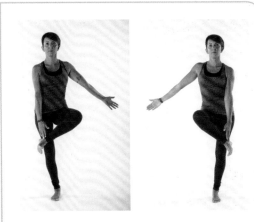

4. HEEL TAP

Stand on your right leg. Lift your left leg up, bend it and turn your knee out. Tap your left heel with your right hand. Switch from leg to leg.

5. TOY SOLDIER

Stand on your right leg and swing your left leg through. Repeat, moving forwards like a toy soldier with straight legs. Start with low legs, but lift each leg higher after a few steps.

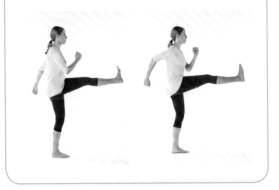

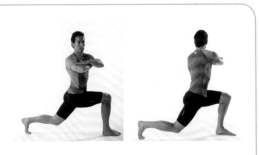

6. THE WALKING LUNGE WITH TWIST

Fold your arms across your chest. Take a large step forwards with your right leg into the lunge and twist your upper body to the right. Step up with the left leg. Continue to travel forwards alternating legs.

10 Post-Baseball and Softball Stretches

Hold each stretch for 20–30 seconds

1. CLASPED HANDS NECK STRETCH

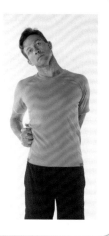

Take your hands behind your back. Interlink them and slide them around to the right side of your waist. Tip your head over to the right. Repeat on the other side.

2. POSTERIOR SHOULDER STRETCH

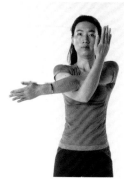

Stand with your left arm straight and at chest height. Place your right arm behind your left elbow and draw the arm across your body. Do not rotate the torso. Repeat on the other side.

3. TRICEPS STRETCH

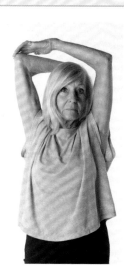

Stand with your feet hip-width apart. Reach up with your right arm and bend it so your hand drops behind your upper back. Use your left hand to gently draw your right elbow back. Repeat on the other side.

4. OVERHEAD STRAP STRETCH

Stand with your feet hip-width apart. Raise your strap, tie or belt overhead with your hands wide. Bend your arms until they form a 90-degree angle and draw your elbows back.

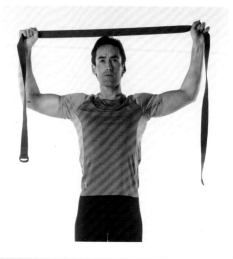

5. CHEST AND SHOULDER STRETCH

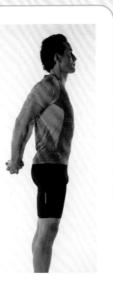

Take your arms behind your back and interlink your hands. Lift your chest, draw your shoulders back and raise your hands. Do not lean forward. Lift your hands higher to go deeper.

6. LOW LUNGE

Lower yourself down to all fours. Step your right foot up in between your hands and raise your upper body. Push your hips forwards. Slowly sink into the lunge.

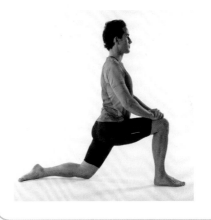

7. KNEELING CALF STRETCH

Shift your body weight back and roll your front foot onto the heel. Point your toes up and/or draw your toes back towards you. To deepen the stretch, hold onto your foot with your right hand and pull gently back. Repeat on the other side.

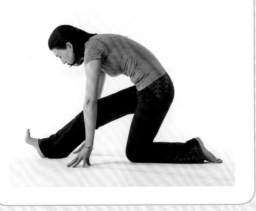

8. BUTTERFLY

Sit down and bring the soles of your feet together. Interlock your hands around your feet or your ankles and sit tall. Lift your chest up in between your arms.

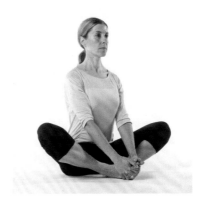

9. BASIC SEATED TWIST

Stretch your legs out in front. Bend your right leg and step it over your left. Wrap your left arm around your leg and hug your leg into your body. Drop your right fingertips behind your back and begin to rotate your torso to the right in stages: lower back, mid back and shoulders and finally turn your head. Repeat on the other side.

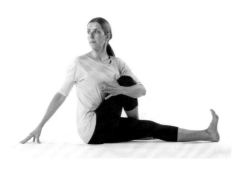

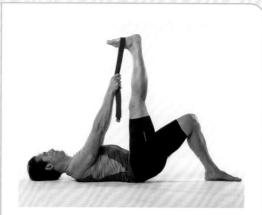

10. HAMSTRING STRAP STRETCH

Lie on your back and loop a strap, belt or tie around the sole of the right foot. Bend your left leg and place the foot on the floor, especially if your hamstrings are tight. Straighten your right leg or bend it a little. Repeat on the other side.

GOING DEEPER: ADVANCED TRICEPS STRETCH

This stretch is particularly aimed at pitchers and bowlers who require excellent range of motion around the shoulder joint. It is also useful in monitoring the flexibility of the pitching/bowling or main throwing arm which is likely to be significantly stiffer than the non-dominant side. Regular stretching will address this shoulder imbalance. As always, never force a stretch and always warm up with some shoulder rolling movements.

Repeat the Triceps stretch with your right arm, but this time take your left arm behind your back and see if you can clasp your hands together. If not, use a strap or tie to bridge the gap.

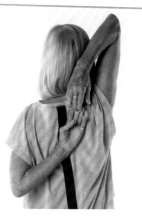

Basketball and Netball

Basketball and netball players must be primed and ready to throw, catch, jump, sprint, twist and move in any direction. These explosive and multi-directional sports require a good level of whole body flexibility particularly around the calves, knees, hamstrings and hips. Basketball players especially are also required to have good foot and ankle strength and a superior sense of balance, hence the inclusion here of some balance-challenging warm-ups. Test your ankle strength by slowing down the Heel and Toe Rocking warm-up technique and try to rise higher onto the balls of the feet. If your feet buckle or sway out to the sides as you rise, practise this movement regularly to reinforce the muscles of the ankles.

6 Warm-Ups for Basketball and Netball

Repeat each stretch x 4

1. SQUEEZE AND SPREAD

Squeeze your hands into fists, tucking the thumb down and hold for five seconds. Now spread your hands wide and hold for five seconds.

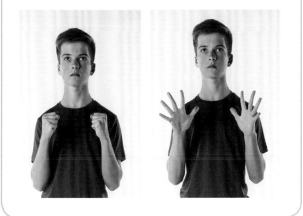

2. HEEL AND TOE ROCKING

Rock your weight back onto the heels and lift your toes off the floor. Rock your weight forwards onto the balls of the feet and lift the heels off the floor.

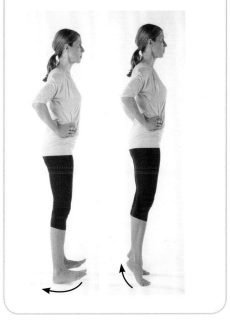

3. SIDE LEG SWING

Stand on your right leg and slowly swing your left leg across your body back and forth. Rest your right hand on a wall for support if required. Repeat on the other side.

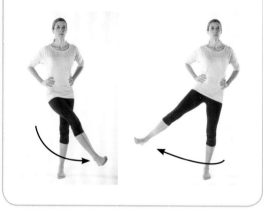

4. SUMO SQUATS

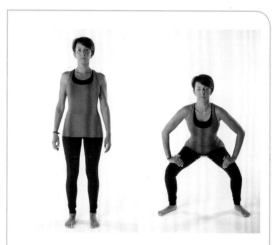

Place your hands on your hips. Step your feet wide with your toes slightly turned outwards. Bend both legs and lower into a squat, checking that your knees are aligned with your toes and your toes are just visible in the squat. Rise back up to standing.

5. SPEED SKATER

Step your feet wider with your toes slightly turned outwards. Lower into a side lunge by bending your right leg and straightening your left. Sweep your left arm across your chest and drop your left elbow down. Let your upper body twist a little. Lunge from side to side.

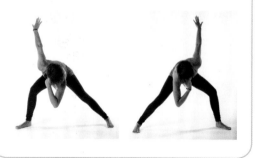

6. WALKING LUNGE WITH TWIST

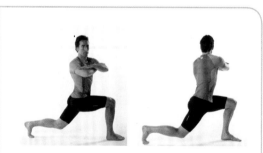

Fold your arms across your chest. Take a large step forwards with your right leg into the lunge and twist your upper body to the right. Step up with the left leg. Continue to travel forwards alternating legs.

10 Post-Basketball and Netball Stretches

Hold each stretch for 20–30 seconds

1. FULL BODY STRETCH

Stand with your feet hip-width apart. Sweep your arms up overhead and interlink your fingers. Press your palms towards the ceiling and remain here, pressing your shoulders downwards.

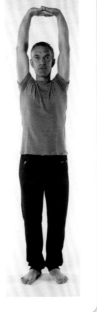

2. FOREARM EXTENSOR STRETCH

Stand with your right arm straight and at shoulder height. Use your left hand to gently push your right hand down. Repeat on the other side.

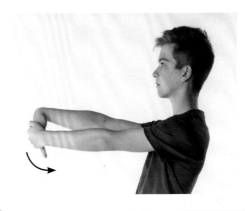

3. FOREARM FLEXOR STRETCH

Stand with your right arm straight and at shoulder height. Use your left hand to gently pull the fingers back. Repeat on the other side.

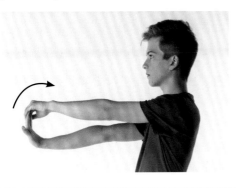

4. POSTERIOR SHOULDER STRETCH

Stand with your right arm straight and at chest height. Place your left hand behind your right elbow and draw your arm across your body. Do not rotate the torso. Repeat on the other side.

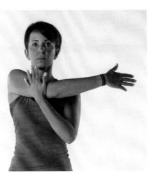

5. STANDING QUAD STRETCH

Either balance on your left leg or place your left hand on a surface for support. Bend your right leg and reach back with your right hand to hold the foot or ankle. Line up your knees and push your hips forwards. Repeat on the other side.

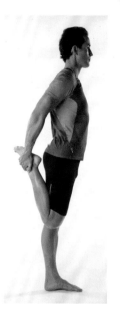

6. WIDE-LEGGED FORWARD BEND

Place your hands on your hips and hinge forwards maintaining a straight spine. Either remain here at a 90-degree angle or lower your fingertips slowly to rest on the ground.

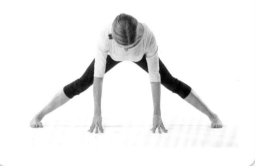

7. ACHILLES SQUAT STRETCH

Stand with your feet hip-width apart. Bend your legs and lower down into a squatting position. Rest your fingertips on the floor in front for balance if necessary.

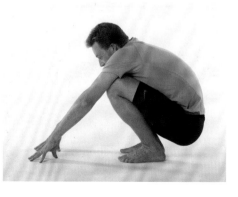

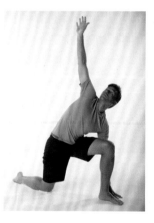

8. LOW LUNGE WITH TWIST

Come down to all fours. Step your left foot up in between your hands. Keep your left hand or fingertips on the floor and sweep your right arm up. Switch legs and sweep your left arm up.

9. SEATED HAMSTRING AND HIP STRAP STRETCH

Bend your right leg and place the sole of your right foot into your inner left thigh. Sit up straight (perch on the edge of a cushion or bend your knees slightly if this is difficult). Loop a strap around your left foot. Remain sitting upright or tilt your upper body forwards without rounding your back. Repeat on the other side.

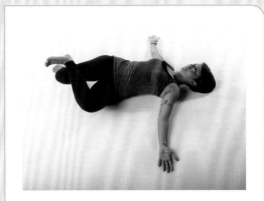

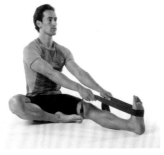

10. HOOKED LYING TWIST

Lie on your back with your legs bent and feet on the floor. Stretch your arms out shoulder-height, palms facing upwards. Lower both legs down to the floor on the left side. Slide your lower leg out and place your foot on top of your higher leg just above your knee.

GOING DEEPER: HIGH LUNGE REVERSE TWIST

This stretch will target all the major muscle groups in the body and improve torso rotation so is ideal for both basketball and netball players. It demands a good level of flexibility in the hamstrings, hips and back.

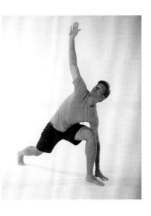

Step your left leg up in between your hands. Shift your weight a little onto your left hand and sweep your right arm up. Either gaze out to the right or up to your top hand. Hold statically for 30-60 seconds, actively reaching up with the top hand while ensuring the hips remain low. Alternatively, to create a dynamic flow, first perform the reverse twist, now switch sides by sweeping your left arm up. Inhale as you reach each arm up and exhale as you return your hand to the floor. Repeat x 4 on each side alternating arms.

Cricket

What stretches cricketers choose will depend on whether they are batting, bowling or fielding. Batters should focus more on the muscles of the head, neck, shoulders and thoracic, or mid back. Bowlers should target the muscles of the shoulders, lower back and hips, while fielders stretch the throwing muscles – the pectorals or chest, shoulders and forearms – and ensure they are ready to run or sprint if required. Having said that, the following routine will suit all cricket players, as all team members will have common tight areas, such as the lower back.

6 Warm-Ups for Cricket

Repeat each stretch x 4

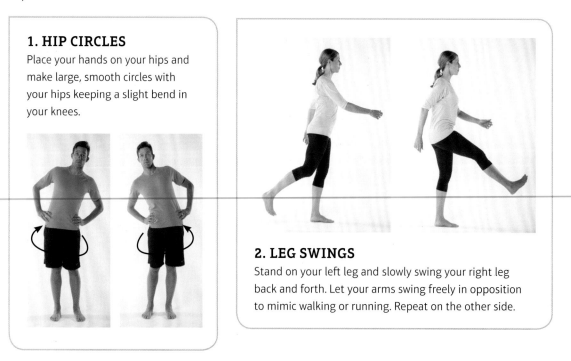

1. HIP CIRCLES
Place your hands on your hips and make large, smooth circles with your hips keeping a slight bend in your knees.

2. LEG SWINGS
Stand on your left leg and slowly swing your right leg back and forth. Let your arms swing freely in opposition to mimic walking or running. Repeat on the other side.

3. BACK KICKS

Stand on your left leg. Bend your left leg and lift your heel to your buttocks. Switch from leg to leg.

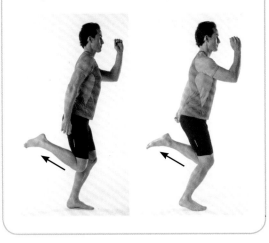

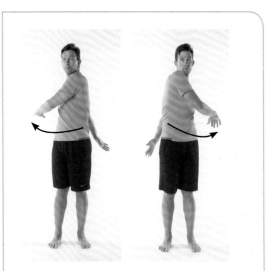

4. STANDING TWIST

Bend your knees and relax your arms by your sides. Twist your upper body to the right and let your arms swing around. Return to the centre and twist to the left. Relax your arms and turn your head and torso as you rotate.

5. SWIMMING ARMS 2

'Swim' your arms mimicking a front crawl movement. Allow your upper body to rotate as you reach forwards with alternate arms. Reverse the exercise by copying the backstroke movement.

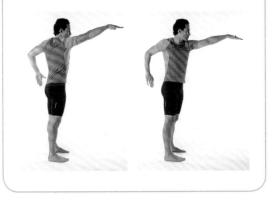

6. WRIST AND HAND WARMER

Interlace your fingers, palms down at chest-height. Pull your hands slightly apart as if your fingers were stuck together until you can feel some traction. Then, alternately flex and extend (bend and draw back) your wrists.

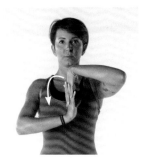

10 Post-Cricket Stretches

Hold each stretch for 20–30 seconds

1. FOREARM FLEXOR STRETCH

Stand with your right arm straight and at shoulder height. Use your left hand to gently pull the fingers back. Repeat on the other side.

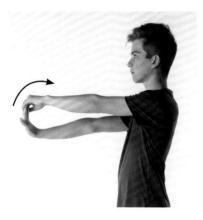

2. POSTERIOR SHOULDER STRETCH

Stand with your left arm straight and at chest height. Place your right arm behind your left elbow and draw your arm across your body. Do not rotate the torso. Repeat on the other side.

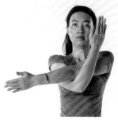

3. TRICEPS STRETCH

Stand with your feet hip-width apart. Reach up with your right arm and bend it so your hand drops behind your upper back. Use your left hand to gently draw your right elbow back. Repeat on the other side.

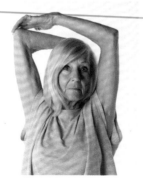

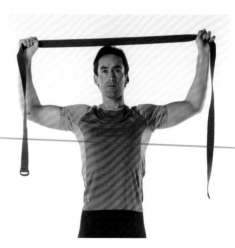

4. OVERHEAD STRAP STRETCH

Stand with your feet hip-width apart. Raise your strap, tie or belt overhead with your hands wide. Bend your arms until they form a 90-degree angle and draw your elbows back.

5. CLASPED HANDS NECK STRETCH

Take your hands behind your back. Interlink them and slide them around the right side of your waist. Tip your head over to the right. Repeat on the other side.

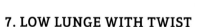

6. HALF PYRAMID STRETCH

Stand with your feet hip-width apart. Step the right leg back and press your heel into the floor. Straighten both legs. Place your hands on your hips and tip forwards maintaining a straight back. Repeat on the other side.

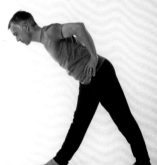

7. LOW LUNGE WITH TWIST

Lower yourself down onto all fours. Step your left foot up in between your hands. Keep your left hand or fingertips on the floor and sweep your right arm up. Switch legs and sweep your right arm up.

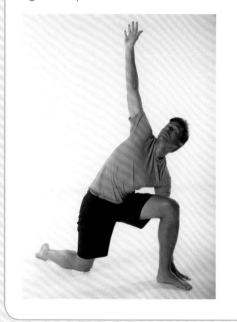

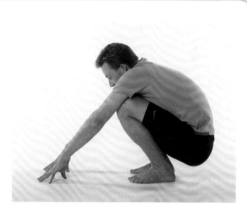

8. ACHILLES SQUAT STRETCH

Stand with your feet hip-width apart and toes facing forwards. Bend your legs and lower down into a squatting position. Rest your fingertips on the floor in front for balance if necessary.

9. SINGLE LEG HUG

Lie on your back and draw your right leg in towards your chest. Keep your left leg straight and press the back of your left knee into the floor. Repeat on the other side.

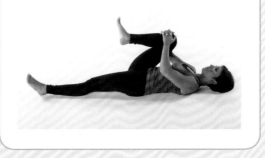

10. BASIC LYING TWIST

Bend both legs and place your feet on the floor. Stretch your arms out shoulder-height, palms facing upwards. Lower both legs down to the floor on the left side and relax them.

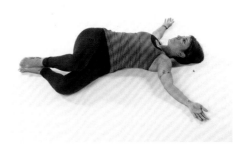

GOING DEEPER: ADVANCED ARM WRAP

Repeated overhead bowling and throwing can cause pain in the rotator cuff area of the shoulder. A preventative measure for bowlers is to focus on stretching the posterior shoulder (or back of shoulder) muscles. This is a deeper version of the Posterior Shoulder Stretch (stretch number 2). It may not be feasible if you have a wide chest or well developed arm/shoulder muscles.

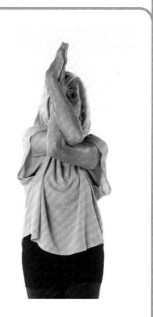

Spread the arms wide at chest height. Wrap your right arm over the left and bend both arms, bringing your forearms closer to your face. If there is space, grip your fingers or hands. Tuck your chin in. Experiment with the following variations:

- Draw your arms downwards
- Lift your arms upwards
- Move your arms to the left
- Move your arms to the right

Unravel and repeat the stretch, crossing the left arm over the right.

Cycling

A little regular stretching can reduce overuse injuries and greatly improve comfort levels in the saddle. The fixed, rounded riding stance is hard on the muscles of the lower and upper back, while hours of repetitive pedalling impacts the hips, thighs and knees. Regular muscle lengthening, particularly of the hamstrings, also has a performance benefit by enabling the rider to adopt an aerodynamic, flatter-backed posture. The Waiter's Bow technique ticks both boxes by maintaining a straight back while lengthening the hamstrings.

6 Warm-Ups for Cyclists

Repeat each stretch x 4

1. HEAD ROLL

Make a continuous semi-circle movement with your head by first tipping your head to the right side by dropping your ear to your shoulder, looking down at your feet, then rolling your head around to your left shoulder. Move in slow motion. Don't tip your head back. Repeat in the other direction.

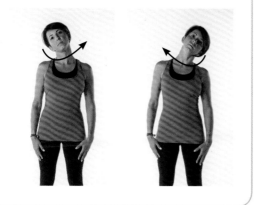

2. KNEE CIRCLE

Stand with your feet together. Bend your legs and place your hands on your knees. Make circles with your knees.

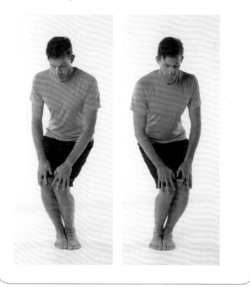

3. BACK KICKS

Stand on your left leg. Bend your right leg as if lifting your heel to your buttocks. Switch from leg to leg.

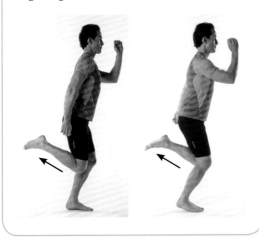

4. LEG SWING

Stand on one leg and slowly swing your other leg back and forth. Let your arms swing freely in opposition to mimic walking or running.

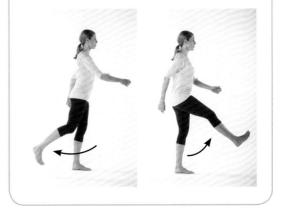

5. LUNGES

Take a step forwards with one leg so that when you bend your front leg to a 90-degree angle, your ankle is over your front knee. Simultaneously drop your back knee down so that it hovers above the floor.

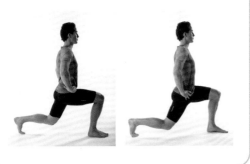

6. HEEL TAP

Stand on your right leg. Lift your left leg up, bend it and turn your knee out. Tap your left heel with your right hand. Switch from leg to leg.

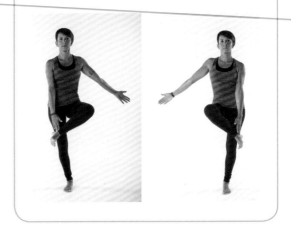

10 Post-Cycling Stretches

Unless otherwise stated hold all stretches for 20-30 seconds.

1. SHOULDER BLADE SQUEEZE

Position your arms in a 'W' shape. Draw your arms back and squeeze your shoulder blades together. Release and bring your forearms closer or touching together. *Repeat x 4.*

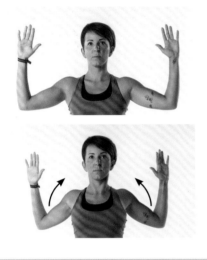

2. ARM WRAP STRETCH

Stand tall. Wrap your arms around your shoulders as if giving yourself a hug. Draw your shoulders away from your ears.

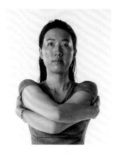

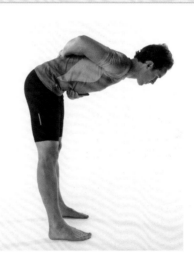

3. ASSISTED NECK EXTENSOR STRETCH

Stand tall. Interlink your hands behind your head. Drop your head forward.

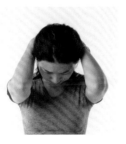

Do not push your head further, but just let your elbows drop forwards so the weight of your arms increases the stretch.

4. WAITER'S BOW

Place your right hand behind your lower back and feel the dip or curve. Place your left palm on your abdomen and begin to tip forwards from your hips while maintaining the dip of your lower back. Exit by bending your knees and pulling in your stomach and rising up to a standing position.

5. ALL FOURS MID-BACK TWIST

Move to all fours, but with your knees wide apart. Ensure your hands are directly under your shoulders. Place your left fingertips on your left shoulder. Stay looking down. As you inhale, point your left elbow up to the ceiling. As you exhale, point your left elbow under your right armpit. *Repeat x 4.*

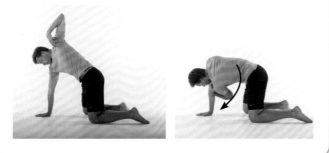

6. KNEELING BACK STRETCH WITH HOOKED THUMBS

From all fours, lower down to sit on your heels. Reach your arms to the top of your mat. Spread your fingers and press down. Hook your thumbs together. Draw your hips away in the opposite direction.

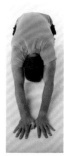

7. LOW LUNGE WITH SIDE BEND

Come down to all fours. Step your right foot up in between your hands and raise your upper body. Tuck your pelvis under. Slowly sink forwards and down into the lunge. Reach high with your left arm and lean your upper body over to the right. Repeat on the other side.

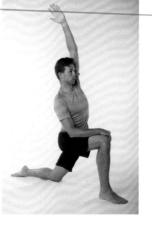

8. LIZARD

From all fours, step your left foot up to the outside of your left hand. Let your hips sink down. Either remain here with straight arms or slowly lower down onto your forearms. A block or book under each forearm will raise the floor level if this proves difficult. Repeat on the other side.

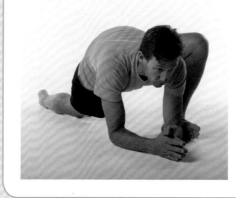

9. FIGURE FOUR

Lie on your back with your legs bent. Lift your right foot off the floor and turn your knee out. Rest your right ankle on top of your left thigh. Either remain here or lift both feet off the floor and draw both legs in towards you. Hold either behind your front thigh or clasp your front shin. If your head tilts back, elevate it on blocks or cushions.

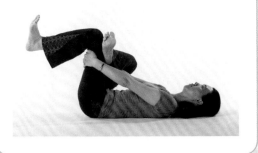

10. LYING STRAP CALF STRETCH

Lie on your back and loop a strap around the sole of the right foot. Straighten your right leg. Bend your left leg and place the foot on the floor. Move your strap higher onto the ball of your foot. Push your heel up.

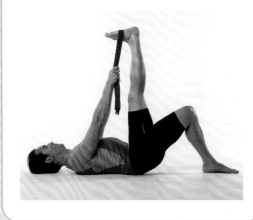

GOING DEEPER: LOW LUNGE WITH QUAD STRETCH

If you are comfortable bearing weight on your back knee, try performing a low lunge combined with a quad stretch. Please note: you will require flexibility to sink your hips low enough so that most of the weight on your back knee is just above the joint, not squarely on your kneecap. Pad your back knee with a cushion or block if required.

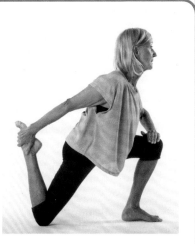

Perform the low lunge with your left foot in front. Lean a little to the left, and bend your right leg. Reach around to hold the right foot. Shift your weight back to the centre and lift your upper body. Either hold still or do the following steps:

- Press the front of your foot into your hand
- Draw your heel closer to your body.

Golf

The golf swing requires excellent flexibility particularly during the upswing phase where the player positions his body for the downswing and follow through. Good mobility is needed in hips, shoulders and especially the thoracic or mid back region which often becomes stiffer as we age. This warm-up and post-play sequence contains plenty of techniques that mimic the golf swing and increase mobility in the spine as well as stretches for the shoulders, hamstrings and lower back.

6 Warm-Ups for Golfers

Repeat each stretch x 4

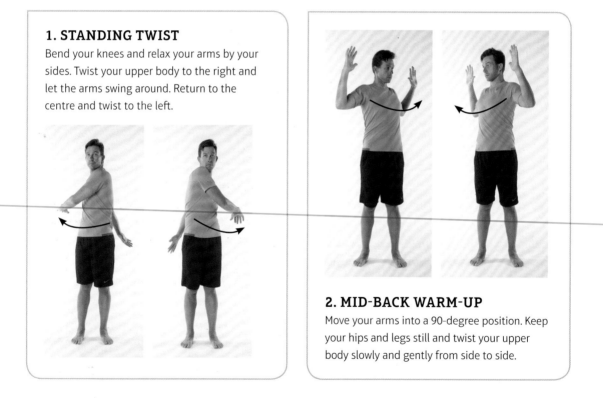

1. STANDING TWIST

Bend your knees and relax your arms by your sides. Twist your upper body to the right and let the arms swing around. Return to the centre and twist to the left.

2. MID-BACK WARM-UP

Move your arms into a 90-degree position. Keep your hips and legs still and twist your upper body slowly and gently from side to side.

3. STRAP SHOULDER LOOSENER

Hold a strap or tie overhead with your hands wide apart and play with the following movements:

- Drop your hands forwards so the strap is in front of your chest.
- Lift the strap overhead so it is behind your head.

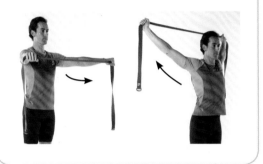

4. HIP CIRCLE

Place your hands on your hips and make large, smooth circles with your hips keeping a slight bend in your knees.

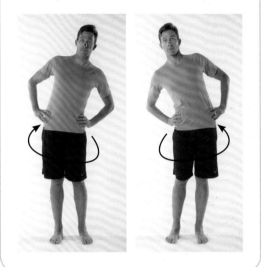

5. LEG SWING

Stand on your left leg and slowly swing your right leg back and forth. Let your arms swing freely in opposition to mimic walking or running.

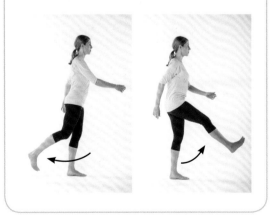

6. TRAVERSING LUNGE WITH TWIST

Fold your arms across your chest. Take a large step forwards with your right leg into the lunge and twist your upper body to the right. Step up with the left leg. Continue to travel forwards alternating legs.

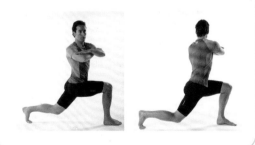

10 Post-Golf Stretches

Hold each stretch for 20–30 seconds

1. TRICEPS STRETCH

Stand with your feet hip-width apart. Reach up with your right arm and bend it so your hand drops behind your upper back. Use your left hand to gently draw your right elbow back. Repeat on the other side.

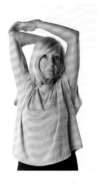

2. POSTERIOR SHOULDER STRETCH

Stand with your left arm straight and at chest height. Place your right arm behind your left elbow and draw your arm across your body. Do not rotate the torso. Repeat on the other side.

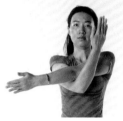

3. OVERHEAD STRAP STRETCH

Stand with your feet hip-width apart. Raise your strap, tie or belt overhead with your hands wide. Bend your arms until they form a 90-degree angle and draw your elbows back.

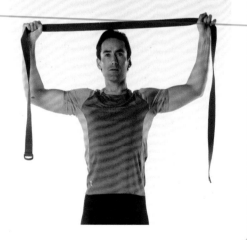

4. CHEST AND SHOULDER STRETCH

Take your arms behind your back and interlink your hands. Lift your chest, draw your shoulders back and raise your hands. Do not lean forward. Lift your hands higher to go deeper.

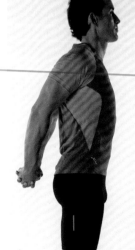

5. FULL BODY SIDE BEND

Stand with your feet hip-width apart. Sweep your arms up overhead and interlink your fingers. Now, simply lean to the side aiming not to tip forwards or backwards. To go deeper, try clasping the top wrist and side bending further.

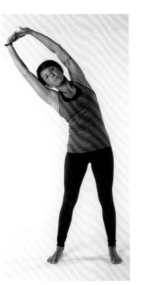

6. HIGH LUNGE

Stand with your feet hip-width apart and your hands on your hips. Take a large step back with your right foot and press your back heel down. Bend your right knee a little and push your hips forwards. Repeat on the other side.

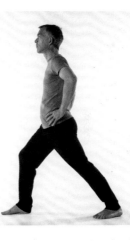

7. ALL FOURS MID-BACK TWIST

Move to all fours, but with your knees wide apart. Ensure your hands are directly under your shoulders. Place your left hand on your left shoulder. Stay looking down. As you inhale, point your left elbow up to the ceiling. As you exhale, point your elbow under your right armpit. *Repeat on the other side.*

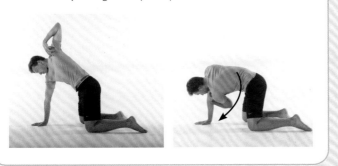

8. KNEELING BACK STRETCH

Move your knees back under your hips and sit on your heels. Reach your arms out in front of you. Position your hands shoulder-width apart. Spread your fingers and press down. Tuck your chin in and rest your forehead on the floor or on a cushion or foam block.

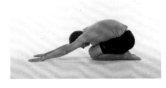

9. BASIC LYING TWIST

Drop your feet to the floor. Stretch your arms out shoulder-height, palms facing upwards. Lower both legs down to the floor on the left side and relax them. Repeat on the other side.

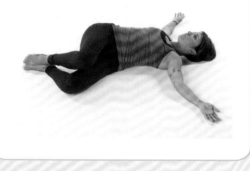

10. STRAP HAMSTRING STRETCH

End the sequence by lying on your back and looping a strap, belt or tie around the sole of the right foot. Bend the left leg and place the foot on the floor, especially if your hamstrings are tight. Straighten the right leg or bend it a little. Repeat on the other side.

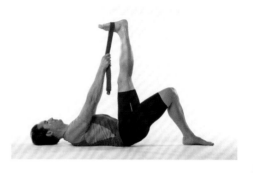

GOING DEEPER: ADVANCED LYING TWIST 1

This advanced stretch can be performed with or without a strap by holding on to the big toe of the extended leg. It ticks a lot of boxes for golfers by improving mobility in the upper body while stretching the hamstrings and outer hip. If it is hard to straighten the leg, just perform the Basic Lying Twist with both legs bent.

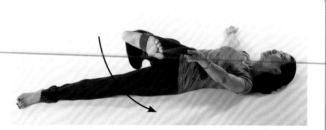

Lie on your back and loop a strap, tie or belt around your right foot. Straighten the leg or leave a small bend. Take hold of both parts of the strap in the left hand and stretch your right arm out along the floor. Move your right leg across your body in slow motion. The stretch should creep up from the ankle, outer calf and iliotibial band all the way to the buttocks. Stop where you feel the deepest stretch. Repeat with the left leg. Take your time (1-3 minutes). This stretch should not be rushed.

Hiking and Walking

Hikers and walkers should focus on warming up the muscles of the ankles, calves and hamstrings and incorporate some balance training especially if traversing rough or uneven ground, to strengthen the lower leg muscles and reduce the likelihood of sprained ankles. The post-hike sequence provides plenty of opportunities to elevate the feet after a hard day's walking by lying on the floor with the legs up. This sequence also eases tension in the lower back, an area that can feel tight and compressed after hiking and walking, especially if you've been trekking with a backpack. Move gently into the foot stretches or omit them if the stretches feel uncomfortable or cause pain.

6 Warm-Ups for Hikers and Walkers   *Repeat each stretch x 4*

1. HEEL AND TOE ROCKING

Rock your weight back into the heels and lift your toes off the floor. Rock your weight forwards onto the balls of the feet and lift the heels off the floor.

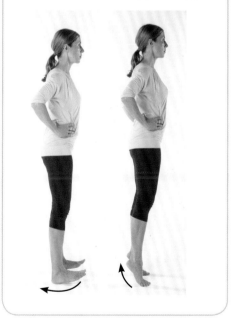

2. ANKLE ROLL

Place your hands on your hips. Stand on your left leg and lift your right foot off the floor. Rotate your foot slowly. Switch feet.

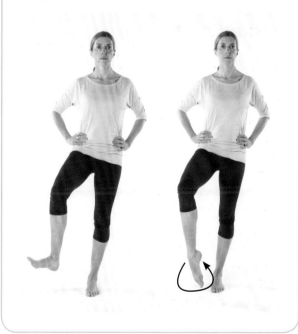

3. LEG SWING

Stand on your left leg and slowly swing your right leg back and forth. Let your arms swing freely in opposition to mimic walking or running.

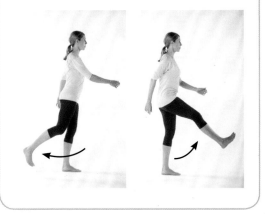

4. BACK KICKS

Stand on your left leg. Bend your right leg as if lifting your heel to your buttocks. Switch from leg to leg.

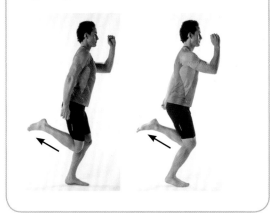

5. MARCHING

Perform a marching action by lifting your knees high. Position your arms in a right angle shape and swing them back and forth.

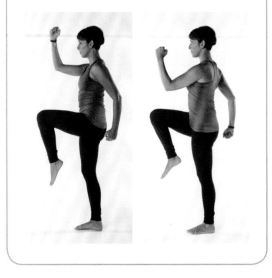

6. STANDING TWIST

Bend your knees and relax your arms by your sides. Twist your upper body to the right and let the arms swing around. Return to the centre and twist to the left. Relax your arms and turn your head and torso as you rotate.

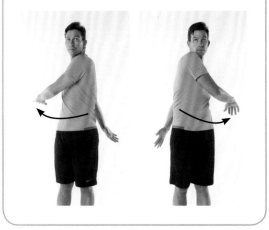

10 Post-Hiking and Walking Stretches

Hold each stretch for 20–30 seconds

1. FULL BODY STRETCH

Stand with your feet hip-width apart. Sweep your arms up overhead and interlink your fingers. Press your palms towards the ceiling.

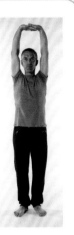

2. STANDING QUAD STRETCH

Either balance on your left leg or place your left hand on a surface for support. Bend your right leg and reach back with your right hand to hold the foot or ankle. Line up your knees and push your hips forwards. Repeat on the other side.

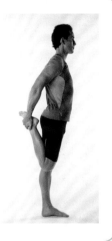

3. LEAN FORWARD STRETCH

Take a small step back with your left leg. Bend your left leg and tip your upper body forwards, placing both hands on your right thigh. Press the sole of your left foot into the floor. Repeat on the other side.

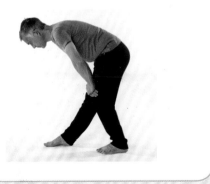

4. LOW LUNGE WITH CHEST STRETCH

Lower yourself down to all fours. Step your right foot up in between your hands and raise your upper body. Push your hips forwards and slowly sink into the lunge. Take your hands behind your back and interlink your fingers. Draw your shoulders back and squeeze your shoulder blades a little closer. Look ahead. Repeat on the other side.

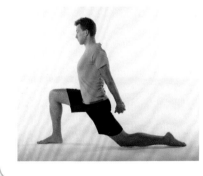

5. KNEELING SOLE STRETCH ON ALL FOURS

Return to all fours. Turn your toes under to feel a stretch on the soles of your feet. Either remain here or walk your hands backwards until you are sitting back on your heels.

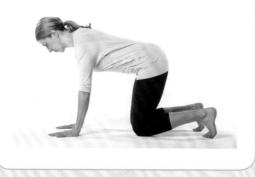

6. KNEELING TOWEL STRETCH

To gain a deeper stretch for the front of the foot and ankle, perform the kneeling position but with a small folded towel, T-shirt or jumper underneath your toes.

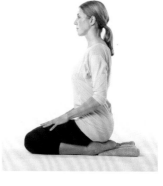

7. BUTTERFLY

Sit down and place the soles of your feet together. Either interlock your hands around your feet or your ankles and sit taller. Lift your chest up between your arms.

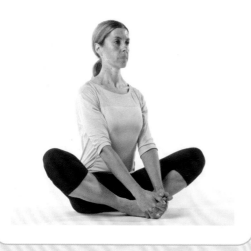

8. LYING CALF STRAP STRETCH

Lie on your back and loop a strap around the sole of your right foot. Push your heel up. Remain still or slowly move your heel from side to side. Repeat on the other side.

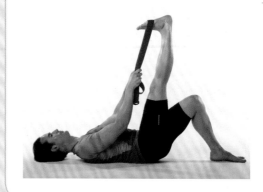

9. LYING INNER THIGH STRAP STRETCH

Hold both parts of your strap in your right hand. Bend your left leg and let your knee drop out to the side to act as a counterbalance. Move your right leg out to the right side to stretch the inner thigh. Repeat on the other side.

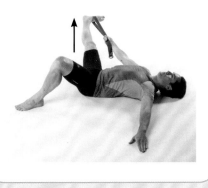

10. LYING OUTER THIGH STRAP STRETCH

Move your right leg back to the centre and hold both parts of the strap in your left hand. Begin to take the right leg slowly across to the left. Stretch your right arm out at shoulder height. Repeat on the other side.

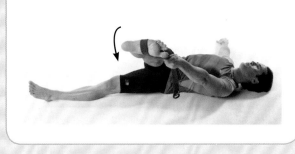

GOING DEEPER: KNEELING SOLE STRETCH

This is a deep stretch for the soles of the feet that would also suit runners. It is also a 'pre-hab' or preventative stretch for plantar fasciitis – inflammation of connective tissue on the bottom of the foot. It does require a good degree of foot flexibility and the ability to kneel comfortably.

Start in an all fours position. Ensure your toes are tucked under and spread wide, then begin to slowly walk your hands backwards and up your thighs until you are sitting on the balls of your feet with a straight back. Remember: for a gentler option, you can stop at a halfway point if you prefer with your hands still on the floor.

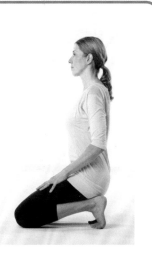

Hockey (Ice and Field)

A hockey player's lower back must be well conditioned – both strong and supple – to comfortably hold the bent-over stance adopted for large periods of the game. The muscles linked to the lower back, such as the hamstrings, also need regular stretching as do the hips, inner thighs and hamstrings. Performance-wise, a player with a good joint range of motion will be able to extend further to reach the ball and is less likely to sustain classic hockey muscular injuries such as groin strain or a torn hamstring.

6 Warm-Ups for Hockey Players

Repeat each stretch x 4

1. DYNAMIC SIDE BENDING

Stand with your feet hip-width. Sweep your left arm up and tip over to the right, trying not to lean forwards or backwards. Return to the centre. Sweep the right arm up and tip to the left.

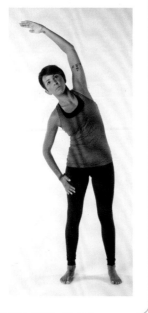

2. SWIMMING ARMS 2

'Swim' your arms mimicking a front crawl movement. Allow your upper body to rotate as you reach forwards with alternate arms. Reverse the exercise by copying the backstroke movement.

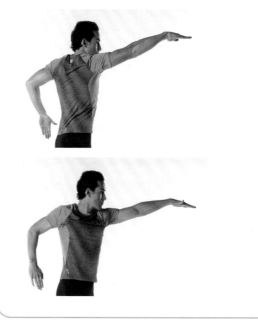

3. HIP CIRCLE

Place your hands on your hips and make large, smooth circles with your hips keeping a slight bend in your knees.

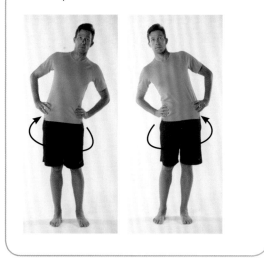

4. SIDE LEG SWING

Stand on your right leg and slowly swing your left leg across your body back and forth. Rest your right hand on a wall for support if required. Repeat on the other side.

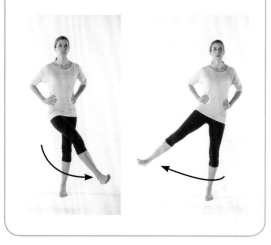

5. LUNGE WITH TWIST

Prepare to lunge, but fold your arms and hold on to your elbows. Position your arms at chest height. As you step forwards with your right foot, rotate only your upper body to the right. Rotate your upper body to face forwards and rise back up to a standing position. Repeat on the other side.

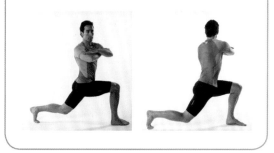

6. SPEED SKATER

Step your feet wide with your toes slightly turned outwards. Lower into a side lunge by bending your right leg and straightening your left. Sweep your left arm across your chest and drop your left elbow down. Let your upper body twist a little. Switch from side to side.

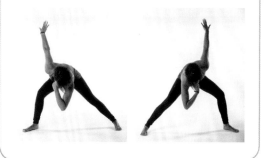

10 Post-Hockey Stretches

Hold each stretch for 20–30 seconds

1. ASSISTED NECK EXTENSOR STRETCH

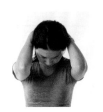

Stand tall. Interlink your hands behind your head. Drop your head, tuck your chin in and let your elbows drop forwards so the weight of the arms increases the stretch.

2. STANDING CROSSED-LEG STRETCH

Stand with your feet hip-width apart. Step your left foot over your right so your legs cross and lean to the right. To deepen this stretch, reach your left arm over by your ear. Repeat on the other side.

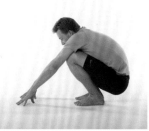

3. LOW LUNGE WITH CHEST STRETCH

Lower yourself down to all fours. Step your right foot up in between your hands and raise your upper body. Push your hips forwards and slowly sink into the lunge. Take your hands behind your back and interlink your fingers. Draw your shoulders back and squeeze your shoulder blades a little closer. Look ahead. Repeat on the other side.

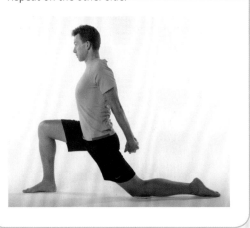

4. ACHILLES SQUAT STRETCH

Stand with your feet hip-width apart and toes facing forwards. Bend your legs and lower down into a squatting position. Rest your fingertips on the floor in front for balance if necessary.

5. BUTTERFLY

Sit down and place the soles of your feet together. Either interlock your hands around your feet or around your ankles and sit taller. Lift your chest up in between your arms.

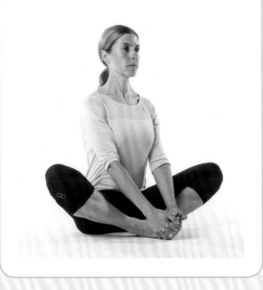

6. SEATED HAMSTRING AND HIP STRAP STRETCH

Bend your right leg and place the sole of your right foot into your inner left thigh. Sit up straight. Loop a strap around your left foot. Remain sitting upright or tilt your upper body forwards without rounding your back. Repeat on the other side.

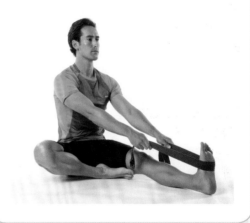

7. COBRA

Lie on your front with your hands just under your shoulders. Press into your hands and slowly raise your upper body off the ground. Lower yourself down and sit back on your heels.

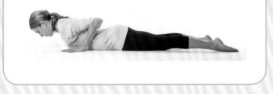

8. DOUBLE LEG HUG

Lie on your back and hug both legs into your abdomen. Rock a little from side to side across the lower back.

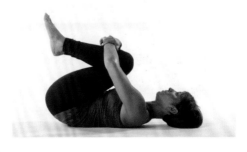

9. FIGURE FOUR SITTING

Sit on the floor with your legs bent. Lift your right foot off the floor and turn your knee out. Rest your right ankle on top of your left thigh. Either stay here or lift both feet off the floor and draw both legs in towards you. Hold behind the front thigh or clasp the front shin. Repeat on the other side.

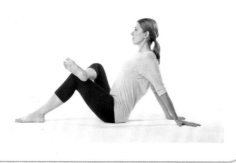

10. BASIC LYING TWIST

Bend both legs and place your feet on the floor. Stretch your arms out at shoulder height, palms facing upwards. Lower both legs down on the floor on the left side and relax them. Repeat on the other side.

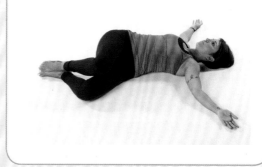

GOING DEEPER: COSSACK STRETCH

This stretch will create supple hamstrings and inner thigh muscles to facilitate deep forwards and sideways lunges for the ball, and also lengthen the calves. It requires balance plus the ability to flex or bend your knees deeply so won't suit a player with stiff or injured knees.

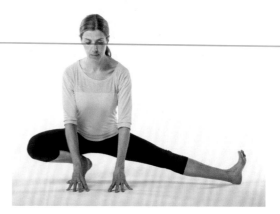

Step your legs wide with your toes slightly turned outwards. Bend your right leg and slowly lower all the way to the floor until your buttocks reach your right heel. Now turn your left toes upwards and try to lower the heel you are kneeling on further to the floor. Repeat on the other side.

Kayaking and Canoeing

The body can feel stiff and cramped sitting for long periods in a kayak or canoe. The lower back is under particular pressure not just from prolonged sitting up, but continual twisting during paddling. This warm-up routine will prepare kayaking/canoeing muscles to reduce initial stiffness and, therefore, the chance of injury, and help create a smoother paddle stroke. The post-paddle static stretch sequence is designed to release tightness in the lower back and target the hip flexors, hamstrings, iliotibial band, neck and shoulders.

6 Warm-Up Stretches

Repeat each stretch x 4

1. MID-BACK WARM-UP

Move your arms into a 90-degree position. Keep your hips and legs still and twist your upper body slowly and gently from side to side.

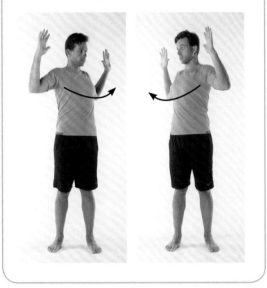

2. SWIMMING ARMS 1

Drop your fingertips onto your shoulders and 'swim' your arms by making alternate circles with your elbows. Roll your shoulders first forwards, then in a backwards motion.

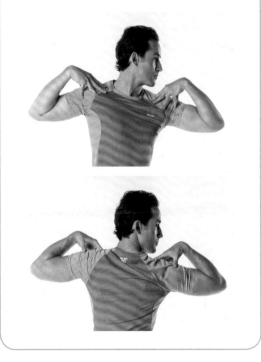

3. HIP CIRCLE

Place your hands on your hips and make large, smooth circles with your hips keeping a slight bend in your knees.

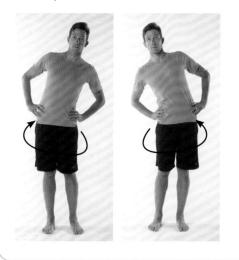

4. LEG SWING

Stand on your left leg and slowly swing your right leg back and forth. Let your arms swing freely in opposition to mimic walking or running. Switch legs.

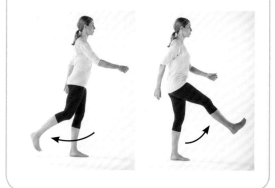

5. HEEL TAP

Stand on your right leg. Lift your left leg up, bend it and turn your knee out. Tap your left heel with your right hand. Switch from leg to leg.

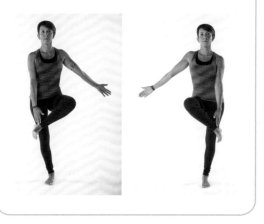

6. DYNAMIC SIDE BENDING

Stand with your feet hip-width apart. Sweep your left arm up and tip over to the right trying not to lean forwards or backwards. Return to the centre. Sweep the right arm up and tip to the left.

10 Post-Kayak and Canoe Stretches

Hold each stretch for 20–30 seconds

1. LATERAL NECK STRETCH

Stand tall with your arms by your sides. Look forwards. Slowly lower your left ear to your left shoulder. To go deeper press your right shoulder downwards. Repeat on the other side.

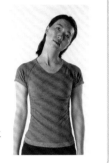

2. STANDING UPPER BACK ROUNDER

Stand with your feet hip-width apart. Round your upper back and tuck your chin in. Reach both arms forwards and interlock your fingers and turn your palms away to face outwards.

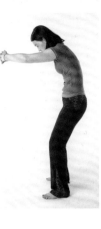

3. STANDING CROSSED-LEG STRETCH

Stand with your feet hip-width apart. Step your left foot over your right so the legs cross. Reach your left arm up and lean to the right. Repeat on the other side.

4. LOW LUNGE WITH CHEST STRETCH

Lower yourself down to all fours. Step your right foot up in between your hands and raise your upper body. Push your hips forwards and sink. into the lunge. Take your hands behind your back and interlink your fingers. Draw your shoulders back and squeeze your shoulder blades a little closer. Look directly ahead. Repeat on the other side.

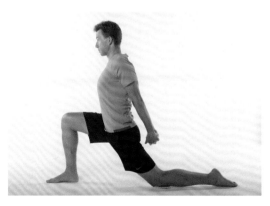

5. SPHINX

Return to all fours. Lie down on your front positioning your elbows directly under your shoulders with your forearms parallel. Draw the shoulder blades slightly closer together.

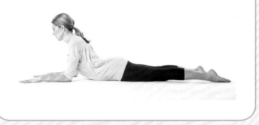

6. KNEELING SIDE STRETCH

Kneel down and lean forward to touch the floor. Walk your hands over to the right. Press the palms into the floor. Hold for 30 seconds. Walk your hands over to the left and press your palms into the floor. *Hold for 30 seconds.*

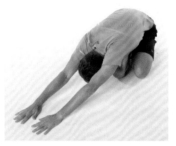

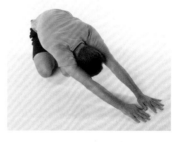

7. SIDE LYING QUAD STRETCH

Lie on your right side with your right leg a little bent under you for balance. Bend your left leg and reach for the foot. Push your hips forward. If you can't reach your foot, loop a strap or tie around it. Repeat on the other side.

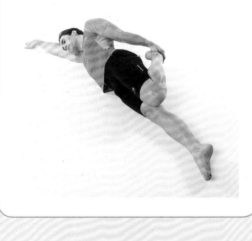

8. DOUBLE LEG HUG

Lie on your back and hug both legs into your abdomen. Rock a little from side to side across the lower back.

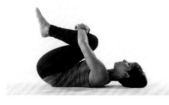

9. BASIC LYING TWIST

Drop your feet to the floor. Stretch your arms out at shoulder height, palms facing upwards. Lower both legs down the floor on the left side and relax them.

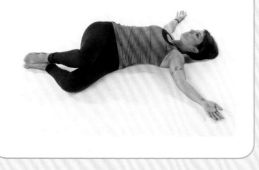

10. HAMSTRING STRAP STRETCH

Lie on your back and loop a strap, belt or tie around the sole of the right foot. Bend the left leg and place the foot on the floor, especially if your hamstrings are tight. Straighten the right leg or keep it a little bent. Repeat on the other side.

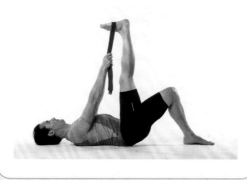

GOING DEEPER: THE LEG KNOT TWIST

This technique will tackle stiff outer hips while giving your back a satisfying twist to wring out the tension accumulated from a morning's seated paddling. You will need the hip and back flexibility to cross your legs and maintain a tall spine. If it is not possible or comfortable to sit with both buttocks on the floor, the hips level and a straight back, try the Basic Seated Twist instead (page 49).

Sit with your legs out straight. Bend your right leg and step it over your left leg. Now lean a

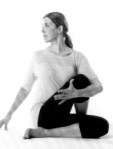

little to the left, bend your left leg and slowly sit back down into the middle space. Sit tall. Wrap your left arm around your right leg and rotate your upper body to the right in stages: lower back, upper back and shoulders and finally turn your head to look over your right shoulder. Every time you breathe in, sit a little taller, every time you breathe out rotate a little more to the right but take care not to strain your back. Unravel the leg and repeat on the other side by stepping your left leg over your right.

Rowing

Rowing works every major muscle group in the body from the legs to the back, arms and shoulders. Flexibility is essential both to maintaining good posture and achieving a long, strong and powerful stroke. A rounded back or 'turtle shell' rowing posture places a strain on the back so it's important to sit tall, or with a neutral spine (the natural slight curve of the lower back in place). The following sequence highlights the hamstrings, gluteals, hip flexors and the calf and ankles while also easing out tension in the back muscles, a common complaint after rowing.

6 Warm-Ups for Rowers

Repeat each stretch x 4

1. LEG SWINGS

Stand on your left leg and slowly swing your right leg back and forth. Let your arms swing freely in opposition to mimic walking or running. Switch legs.

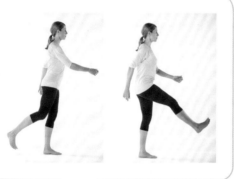

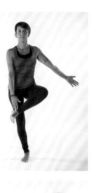

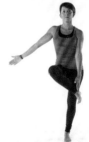

2. BACK KICK

Stand on your left leg. Bend your right leg as if lifting your heel to your buttocks. Switch from leg to leg.

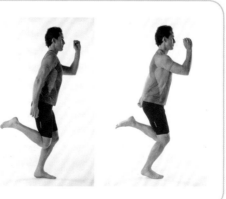

3. HEEL TAP

Stand on your right leg. Lift your left leg up, bend it and turn your knee out. Tap your left heel with your right hand. Switch from leg to leg.

4. MID-BACK WARM-UP

Move your arms into a 90-degree position. Keep your hips and legs still and twist your upper body slowly and gently from side to side.

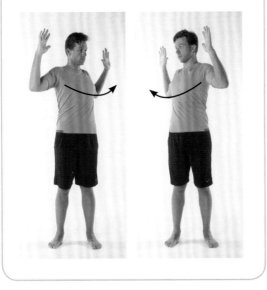

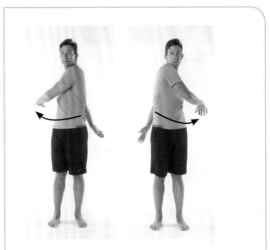

5. STANDING TWIST

Bend your knees and relax your arms by your sides. Twist your upper body to the right and let the arms swing around. Return to the centre and twist to the left. Relax your arms and turn your head and torso as you rotate.

6. SWIMMING ARMS 1

Drop your fingertips onto your shoulders and 'swim' your arms by making alternate circles with your elbows. Roll your shoulders first forwards, then in a backwards motion.

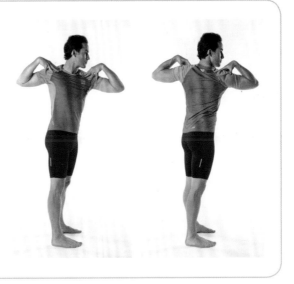

10 Post-Rowing Stretches

Hold each stretch for 20–30 seconds

1. CLASPED HANDS NECK STRETCH

Take your hands behind your back. Interlink them and slide them around the right side of your waist. Tip your head over to the right. Repeat on the other side.

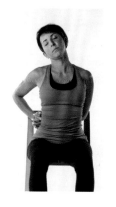

2. POSTERIOR SHOULDER STRETCH

Stand with your right arm straight and at chest height. Place your left arm behind your right elbow and draw your arm across your body. Do not rotate the torso. Repeat on the other side.

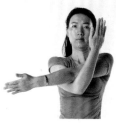

3. CHEST AND SHOULDER STRETCH

Take your arms behind your back and interlink your hands. Lift your chest, draw your shoulders back and raise your hands. Do not lean forward. Lift your hands higher to go deeper.

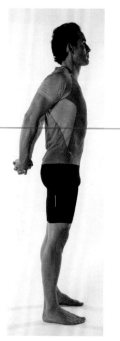

4. STANDING QUAD STRETCH

Either balance on your left leg or place your left hand on a surface for support. Bend your right leg and reach back with your right hand to hold the foot or ankle. Line up your knees and push your hips forwards. Repeat on the other side.

5. WAITER'S BOW

Place your right hand behind your lower back and feel the dip or curve. Place your left palm on your abdomen and begin to tip forwards from your hips while maintaining the dip of your lower back. Exit by bending your knees and pulling in your stomach and rising up to a standing position.

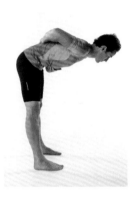

6. LOW LUNGE WITH SIDE BEND

Come down to all fours. Step your right foot up in between your hands and raise your upper body. Tuck your pelvis under. Slowly sink forwards and down into the lunge. Reach high with your left arm and lean your upper body over to the right. Repeat on the other side.

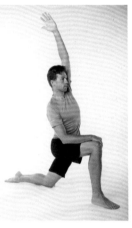

7. KNEELING HAMSTRING AND CALF STRETCH

Perform a Lunge by starting on all fours and stepping your right foot up between your hands. Shift your body weight back and roll your front foot onto the heel. Point your toes up and/or draw your toes back towards you. To deepen the stretch, hold onto your foot with your right hand and pull gently back.

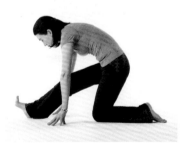

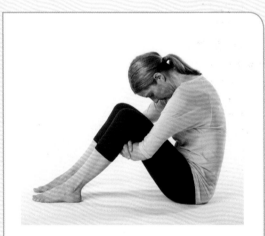

8. THE ROUNDED BACK STRETCH

Sit with your legs bent and feet on the floor. Clasp your hands around the back of your thighs. Round your back, let your head drop down and lean backwards.

9. FIGURE FOUR SITTING

Lie on your back with your legs bent. Lift your right foot off the floor and turn your knee out. Rest your right ankle on top of your left thigh. Stay here or lift both feet off the floor and draw both legs in towards you. Hold behind your front thigh or clasp your front shin. Repeat on the other side.

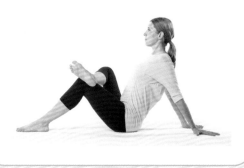

10. HOOKED LYING TWIST

Lie down with your legs bent and feet on the floor. Stretch your arms out at shoulder-height, palms facing upwards. Lower both legs down onto the floor on the left side. Slide your lower leg out and place your foot on top of the higher leg, just above your knee. Repeat on the other side.

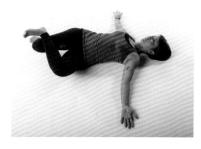

GOING DEEPER: THE RACK

The Rack is a deep shoulder and chest stretch that reverses the crunched forward or 'catch' phase of the rowing stroke. It is a powerful stretch for your shoulders and should be avoided if you have an injury in this region. Having said that, you can make The Rack as strong or gentle as you like simply by moving your hands further away and closer together or nearer and wider apart. Remember to lift your chest to bring in your chest muscles or 'pecs'.

Move to a seated position and straighten your legs. Take your hands behind your back, about body-width apart, with your fingers facing back, and press them into the mat. Lift your

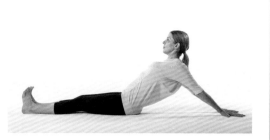

chest, but keep your chin tucked in. Squeeze your shoulder blades together. To go deeper, try again, but with your hands either close together and/or further away. Note: this is a deep stretch for your shoulders so avoid it or only do the first part of the stretch if you have an injury.

Rugby

Rugby is a multi-directional sport requiring players to make sudden lunging, twisting or diving movements. Flexibility, therefore, as well as strength, is crucial to ensure muscles are pliant and ready to respond fast without the risk of injury. The six warm-up techniques reflect this in being dynamic and multi-directional to prepare athletes for the game, while the cool down static stretches target every major muscle group used in rugby and release tension in your back.

6 Warm-Ups for Rugby

Repeat each stretch x 4

1. SWIMMING ARMS 1

Drop your fingertips onto your shoulders and 'swim' your arms by making alternate circles with your elbows. Roll your shoulders first forwards, then in a backwards motion.

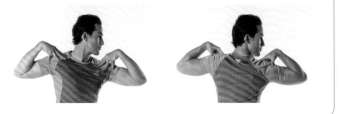

2. SIDE LEG SWINGS

Stand on your left leg and slowly swing your right leg across your body back and forth. Rest your right hand on a wall for support if required. Switch legs.

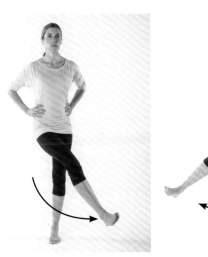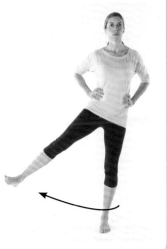

3. TOY SOLDIER

Stand on your right leg and swing your left leg through. Repeat, moving forwards like a toy soldier with straight legs. Start with low legs but lift each leg higher after a few steps.

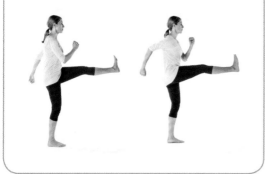

4. BACK KICK WALKING

Walk forwards, kicking your back heel up towards your buttocks. Or, for a more dynamic version, perform Back Kick Walking hopping from leg to leg.

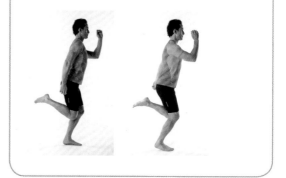

5. TRAVERSING LUNGE WITH TWIST

Fold your arms across your chest. Take a large step forwards with your right leg into the lunge and twist your upper body to the right. Step up with your left leg. Continue to travel forwards alternating legs.

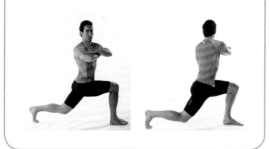

6. TRAVERSING SUMO SQUATS

Do wide Sumo-style side lunges by taking a step out to the side, bending both knees to drop into the squat. Position your toes slightly turned outwards. You should still be able to see your toes as you sit into the squat. Traverse to the right side, then traverse to the left.

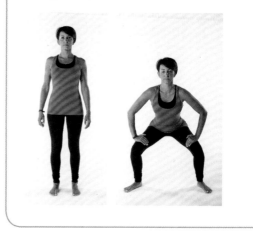

10 Post-Rugby Stretches

Hold each stretch for 20–30 seconds

1. FULL BODY SIDE BEND

Stand with your feet hip-width apart. Sweep your arms up overhead and interlink your fingers. Now lean to the side aiming not to tip forwards or backwards. To go deeper, try clasping your top wrist and side bending further.

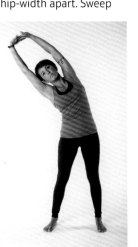

2. TRICEPS STRETCH

Stand with your feet hip-width apart. Reach up with your right arm and bend it so your hand drops behind your upper back. Use your left hand to gently draw your right elbow back.

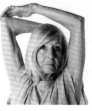

3. WIDE-LEGGED FORWARD BEND

Place your hands on your hips and hinge forwards maintaining a straight spine. Either remain here at a 90-degree angle or lower your fingertips slowly to rest on the ground.

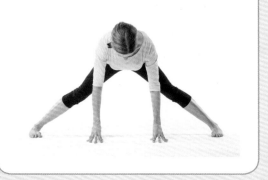

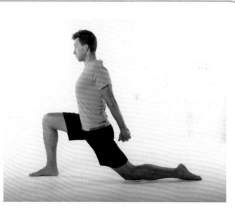

4. LOW LUNGE WITH CHEST STRETCH

Lower yourself down to all fours. Step your right foot up in between your hands and raise your upper body. Slowly sink forwards and down into the lunge and push your hips forwards. Now take your hands behind your back and interlink your fingers. Draw your shoulders back and squeeze your shoulder blades a little closer. Look ahead.

5. ALL FOURS MID-BACK TWIST

Move to all fours, but with your knees wide apart. Ensure your hands are directly under your shoulders. Place your left hand on your left shoulder. Stay looking down. As you inhale, point your left elbow up to the ceiling. As you exhale, point your left elbow under your right armpit. *Repeat x 4.*

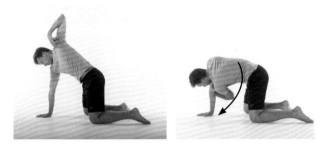

6. KNEELING BACK STRETCH

Lower down to sit on your heels. Reach your arms to the top of your mat. Spread your fingers wide and press down. Now draw your hips away in the opposite direction.

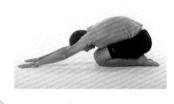

7. BUTTERFLY

Sit down and bring the soles of your feet together. Either interlock your hands around your feet or around your ankles and sit taller. Lift your chest up in between your arms.

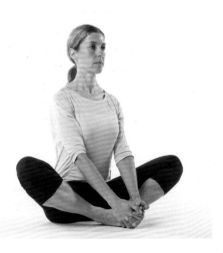

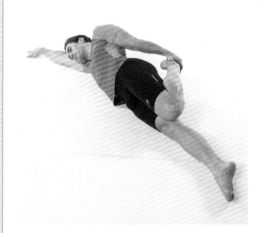

8. SIDE LYING QUAD STRETCH

Lie on your right side with your right leg a little bent under you for balance. Bend your left leg and reach for the foot. Push your hips forward. If you can't reach your foot, loop a strap or tie around it. Repeat on the other side.

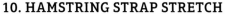

9. FIGURE FOUR

Lie on your back with your legs bent. Lift your right foot off the floor and turn your knee out. Rest your right ankle on top of your left thigh. Either stay here or lift both feet off the floor and draw both legs in towards you. Hold either behind your front thigh or clasp your front shin. If your head tilts back, elevate it on blocks or cushions. Repeat on the other side.

10. HAMSTRING STRAP STRETCH

Lie on your back and loop a strap, belt or tie around the sole of the right foot. Bend your left leg and place your foot on the floor, especially if your hamstrings are tight. Straighten your right leg or bend it a little. Stay for 30 seconds. Now push your heel up and toes down to target your calf and Achilles. Stay for a further 30 seconds.

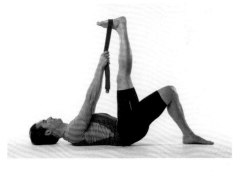

GOING DEEPER: ADVANCED LYING TWIST 1

This advanced stretch can be performed with or without a strap by holding on to the big toe of your extended leg. It will release tension in your upper body while stretching your hamstrings and outer hip. If it is hard to straighten your leg, just perform the Basic Lying Twist with both legs bent.

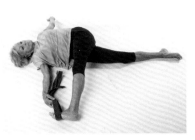

Lie on your back and loop a strap, tie or belt around your right foot. Straighten your leg or leave a small bend. Now take hold of both parts of the strap in your left hand and stretch your right arm out along the floor. Begin to draw your right leg across your body in slow motion. The stretch should creep up from your ankle, outer calf and iliotibial band all the way up to your buttocks. Stop where you feel the deepest stretch. Repeat with your left leg. Take your time (1-3 minutes). This stretch should not be rushed.

Running

Running is a repetitive, forwards-only movement which can result in tightness around the outer hips and thighs, hamstrings, hip flexors and quads. Regular stretching is vital to rebalance these muscle groups, aid recovery and even enhance your running style by encouraging good posture and a relaxed, fluid stride. The following warm-up and cool down techniques also aim to keep the feet supple and responsive on hills or trails and able to weather the impact of running on harder city surfaces.

6 Warm-Ups for Runners

Repeat each stretch x 4

1. HEEL AND TOE ROCKING

Rock your weight back into the heels and lift your toes off the floor. Rock your weight forwards onto the balls of your feet and lift your heels off the floor.

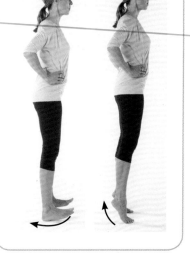

2. SIDE LEG SWINGS

Stand on your left leg and slowly swing your right leg across your body back and forth. Rest your left hand on a wall for support if required. Switch legs.

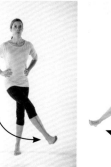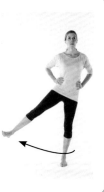

3. HEEL TAPS

Stand on your right leg. Lift your left leg up, bend it and turn your knee out. Tap your left heel with your right hand. Switch from leg to leg.

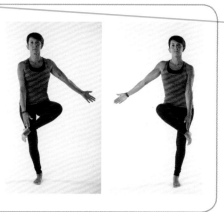

4. TOY SOLDIER

Stand on your right leg and swing your left leg through. Repeat, moving forwards like a toy soldier with straight legs. Start with low legs but lift each leg higher after a few steps.

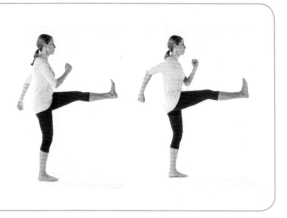

5. BACK KICK WALKING

Walk forwards, kicking your back heel up towards your buttocks. Or, for a more dynamic version, perform Back Kick Walking hopping from leg to leg.

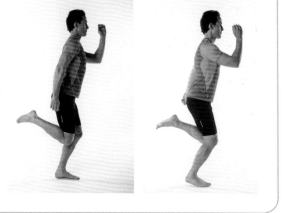

6. TRAVERSING LUNGE

Take a large step forwards with your right leg and drop your left knee downwards so that it hovers above the floor. Step up with the left leg. Continue to travel forwards alternating legs.

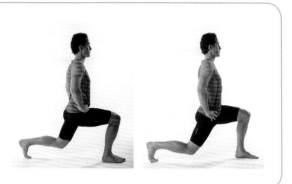

10 Post-Run Stretches

Hold each stretch for 20–30 seconds

1. FULL BODY STRETCH

Stand with your feet hip-width apart. Sweep your arms up overhead and interlink your fingers. Press your palms towards the ceiling.

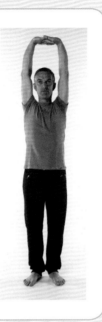

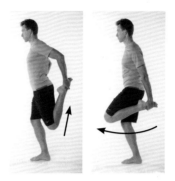

2. DYNAMIC QUAD STRETCH

Stand tall with your feet hip-width apart. Slowly bend your left leg and reach around to hold your foot with your left hand. If required, hold onto a chair for balance. Push your hips forward. Bend your right leg and draw your left leg back further. Now start to move your leg by alternately pointing your knee forward and drawing your knee back. *Repeat x 6 on each side.*

3. HALF PYRAMID STRETCH

Stand with your feet hip-width. Step your left leg back and press your heel into the floor. Straighten both legs. Place your hands on your hips and tip forwards maintaining a straight back. Either remain here or bring your fingertips to the floor.

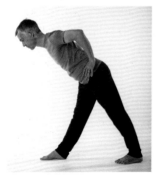

4. WALKING DOG

Start on all fours. Spread your fingers wide. Lift your hips up to make a triangle shape with your body. Bend one leg and push the other heel towards the floor. Continue, moving side to side or pause for 10 seconds on each leg.

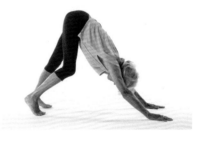

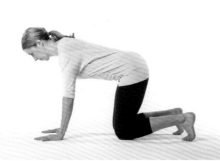

5. KNEELING SOLE STRETCH

Return to all fours. Turn your toes under to feel a stretch on the soles of the feet. Either remain here or walk your hands backwards until you are sitting back on your heels.

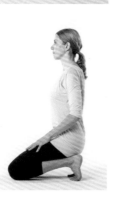

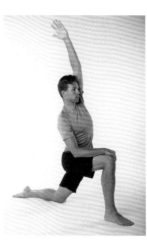

6. LOW LUNGE WITH SIDE BEND

Step your right foot up in between your hands and raise your upper body. Tuck your pelvis under. Slowly sink forwards and down into the lunge. Reach high with your left arm and lean your upper body over to the right.

7. LIZARD

Move into the Lunge position, but position your left foot outside your left hand. Sink your hips deeper into the lunge. Bend your arms or lower onto your forearms. Uncurl your back toes so the front of your foot rests on the floor.

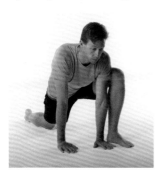

8. PIGEON

Return to all fours. Slide your right knee up behind your right wrist. Wiggle your right foot a little over to the left. Straighten your back leg. Lower yourself slowly onto your forearms. To move deeper, lower your upper body further by resting your forehead on your stacked hands or the floor. Repeat on the other side.

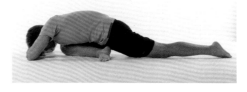

9. LYING INNER THIGH STRAP STRETCH

Lie on the floor with your right leg elevated. Hold both parts of your strap in your right hand. Bend your left leg and let your knee drop out to the side to act as a counterbalance. Now slowly take the right leg out to the right. Repeat on the other side.

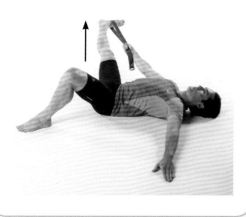

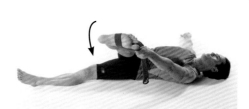

10. LYING OUTER THIGH STRAP STRETCH

Draw your right leg back to the centre and hold both parts of the strap in your left hand. Move your right leg slowly across to the left. Reach your right arm out at shoulder height. Repeat on the other side.

GOING DEEPER: LYING LEG KNOT

If you are a supple runner, try this powerful stretch for the muscles of the outer thighs and hips while recovering on your back. Its accessibility depends on hip flexibility. But I've also found that women seem to find it easier to perform than men. Try holding your toes and pressing them down for an additional front-of-foot stretch.

Lie on your back with your legs bent. Cross your right leg over your left at thigh level and hug both legs in towards you. Hold just below your top knee or clasp both feet. Switch legs by crossing your left leg on top.

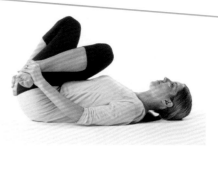

Soccer

Soccer players can run between six and eight miles during a match and alternate between jogging, running and sprinting impacting the feet, calves, groin and hamstrings. Soccer is also a truly multidirectional sport with side lunges, backwards running and jumping. A good warm-up and regular static stretching will ensure a player is supple and primed to respond to the unexpected and stay injury-free throughout the season.

6 Warm-Ups for Soccer

Repeat each stretch x 4

1. HEEL AND TOE ROCKING

Rock your weight back into the heels and lift your toes off the floor. Rock your weight forwards onto the balls of the feet and lift the heels off the floor.

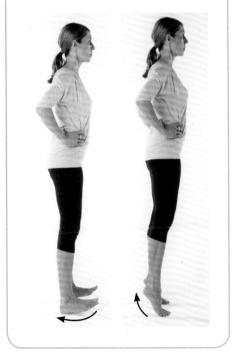

2. MARCHING

March forwards lifting your knees high. Swing your arms back and forth.

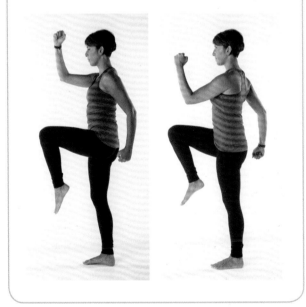

3. TOY SOLDIER

Stand on your right leg and swing your left leg through. Repeat, moving forwards like a toy soldier with straight legs. Start with low legs but lift each leg higher after a few steps.

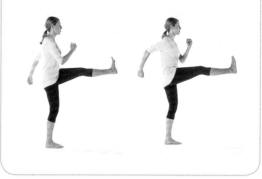

4. BACK KICK WALKING

Walk forwards, kicking your back heel up towards your buttocks. Or, for a more dynamic version, perform Back Kick Walking hopping from leg to leg.

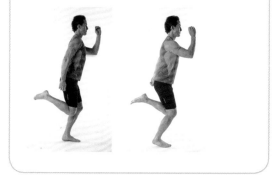

5. TRAVERSING LUNGE

Take a large step forwards with your right leg and drop your back knee so that it hovers above the floor. Step up with your left leg. Continue to travel forwards alternating legs.

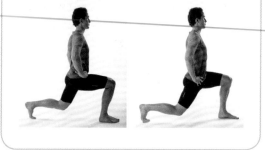

6. TRAVERSING SUMO SQUATS

Take a wide step out to the side, bending both knees to drop into the squat. Position your toes slightly turned outwards. You should be able to still see your toes as you sit into the squat. Traverse to the right side, then traverse to the left.

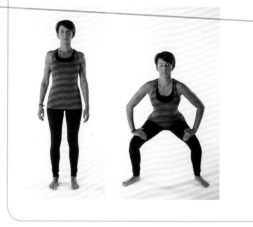

10 Post-Soccer Stretches

Hold each stretch for 20–30 seconds

1. STANDING CROSSED-LEG STRETCH

Stand with your feet hip-width. Step your left foot over your right so the legs cross. Reach your left arm up and lean to the right. Repeat on the other side.

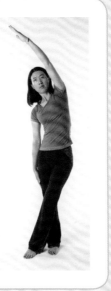

2. STANDING QUAD STRETCH

Either balance on your left leg or place your left hand on a surface for support. Bend your right leg and reach back with your right hand to hold the foot or ankle. Line up your knees and push your hips forwards. To go deeper, bend the standing leg a little and draw the bent leg further back. Repeat on the other side.

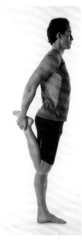

3. DOWNWARD FACING DOG

Start on all fours. Spread your fingers wide. Lift your hips up to make a triangle shape with your body. Press both heels down towards the floor.

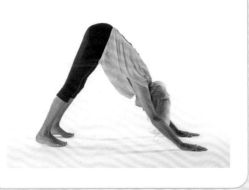

4. LOW LUNGE

Lower yourself down to all fours. Step your right foot up in between your hands and raise your upper body. Push your hips forward. Slowly lower into the lunge.

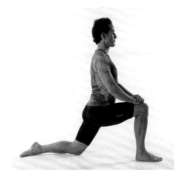

5. FROG

From all fours, move your knees wider and bring your toes to touch. Lower back to sit on your heels. Stack your hands on top of each other and rest your forehead on your hands.

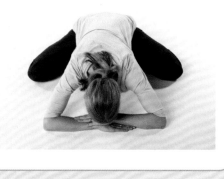

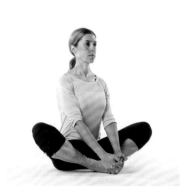

6. BUTTERFLY

Sit either on the floor, or the edge of a cushion or foam block if you find it hard to straighten the spine in this position. Bring the soles of your feet together. Clasp your hands either around your feet or around your ankles and sit tall.

7. BASIC SEATED TWIST

Stretch your legs out in front. Bend your right leg and step it over your left. Wrap your left arm around your leg and draw your leg into your body. Drop your right fingertips behind your back and begin to rotate your torso to the right in stages: lower back, mid back and shoulders and finally your head turns to look to the right.

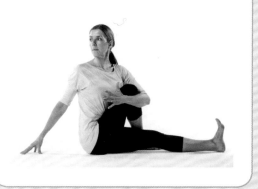

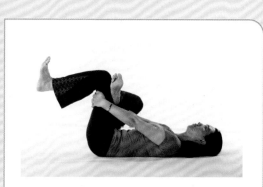

8. FIGURE FOUR

Lie on your back with your legs bent. Lift your right foot off the floor and turn your knee out. Rest your right ankle on top of your left thigh. Either stay here or lift both feet off the floor and draw both legs in towards you. Hold behind your front thigh or clasp your front shin. Repeat on the other side.

9. LYING HAMSTRING STRAP STRETCH

Lie on your back and loop a strap, belt or tie around the sole of your right foot. Bend your left leg and place the foot on the floor, especially if your hamstrings are tight. Straighten your right leg or bend it a little. Repeat on the other side.

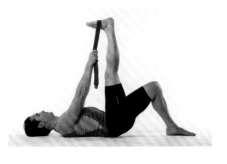

10. LYING CALF STRAP STRETCH

Remain in the Lying Strap Hamstring Stretch, but move your strap higher onto the ball of your foot and push your heel up. Stay still or move your heel slowly from side to side.

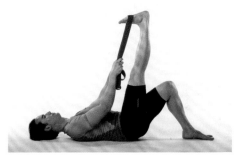

GOING DEEPER: THE LIZARD

The Lizard is basically a very low lunge with a deep groin stretch making it a useful flexibility technique for the more supple player as both groin and hamstring strains are common in soccer. Lizard also stretches the hip flexor of the back leg. Two or more foam yoga or Pilates blocks are useful props for this stretch, but a few thick books will work too. You may also need to pad your back knee with a block or cushion.

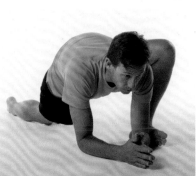

From all fours, step your left foot up to the outside of the left hand. Let your hips sink down and see if you can lower your upper body down onto your forearms. A block or book under each forearm will raise the floor level if this proves difficult. Uncurl your back toes so the front of your foot rests on the floor. Drop your head down and hold. Repeat on the other side.

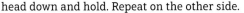

Skiing and Snowboarding

Ten minutes spent stretching out the legs and hips will greatly reduce the muscular aches skiers and snowboarders feel as they exit the slopes at the end of a long day. Neither sport requires great flexibility, but the fixed bent-legged stance can create achy calves, shins, thighs, hamstrings and buttocks. Rebalancing this tightness through muscle lengthening will leave skiers and snowboarders feeling fresh and ready to return to the slopes.

6 Warm-Ups for Skiers and Snowboarders

Repeat each stretch x 4

1. HEEL AND TOE ROCKING

Rock your weight back into the heels and lift your toes off the floor. Rock your weight forwards onto the balls of the feet and lift the heels off the floor.

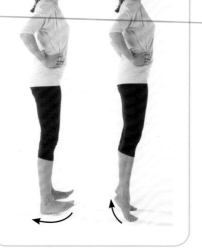

2. HIP CIRCLE

Place your hands on your hips and make large, smooth circles with your hips keeping a slight bend in your knees.

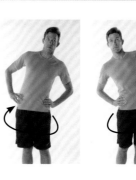

3. STANDING TWIST

Bend your knees and relax your arms by your sides. Twist your upper body to the right and let the arms swing around. Return to the centre and twist to the left. Relax your arms and turn your head and torso as you rotate.

4. BACK KICK

Stand on your left leg with your hands in front of you.
Bend your right leg as if lifting your heel to your buttocks.
Switch from leg to leg.

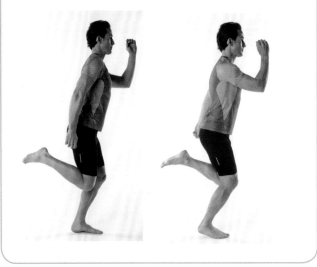

5. SPEED SKATER

Step your feet wider with your toes
slightly turned outwards. Lower
into a side lunge by bending your
right leg and straightening your
left. Sweep your left arm across
your chest and drop your left elbow
down. Let your upper body twist a
little. Switch from side to side.

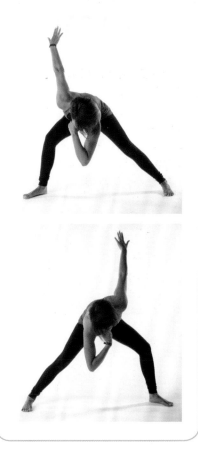

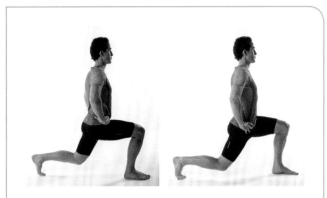

6. TRAVERSING LUNGE

Take a large step forwards with your right leg and drop
your left knee downwards so that it hovers above the
floor. Step up with the left leg. Continue to travel forwards
alternating legs.

10 Post-Ski and Snowboard Stretches

Hold each stretch for 20–30 seconds

1. STANDING BACK BEND

Place your hands on your lower back, fingers pointing downwards. Stay looking forward or slightly down. Lean back. Push your hips forward. Draw your elbows together.

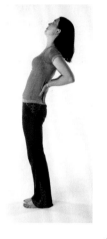

2. HALF PYRAMID OR FULL PYRAMID STRETCH

Straighten both legs. Place your hands on your hips and tip forwards maintaining a straight back. Remain here or bring your fingertips to the floor either side of your front foot.

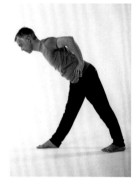

3. LOW LUNGE WITH SIDE BEND

From the Low Lunge, reach high with your left arm and lean the upper body over to the right. *Hold for 20 seconds.* Repeat on the other side. *Hold for 20 seconds.*

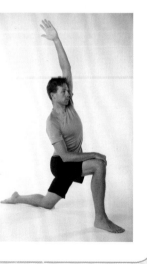

4. LOW LUNGE

Lower yourself down to all fours. Step your right foot up in between your hands and raise your upper body. Push your hips forwards. Slowly sink down into the lunge.

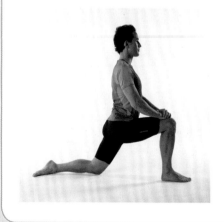

5. KNEELING CALF STRETCH

Shift your body weight back and roll your front foot onto the heel. Point your toes up and draw your toes back towards you. To deepen the stretch, hold onto your foot with your right hand and pull gently back.

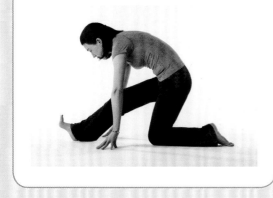

6. KNEELING TOWEL STRETCH

To gain a deeper stretch for the front of the foot and ankle, perform the kneeling position, but with a small folded towel or jumper underneath your toes.

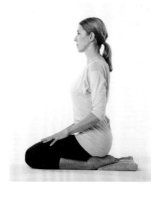

7. BUTTERFLY

Sit down and bring the soles of your feet together. Either interlock your hands around your feet or around your ankles and sit taller. Lift your chest up in between your arms.

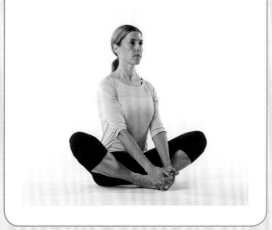

8. FIGURE FOUR CHAIR

Sit on a chair with a straight back and both feet on the floor. Lift your left foot off the floor and turn your knee out. Rest your left ankle on top of your right thigh. Keeping your back straight, lean your upper body forwards a little. Lean further forwards to increase the intensity of the stretch. Repeat on the other side.

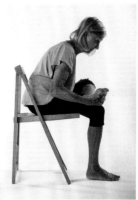

9. BASIC SEATED TWIST

Stretch your legs out in front. Bend your right leg and step it over your left. Wrap your left arm around your leg and draw your leg into your body. Drop your right fingertips behind your back and begin to rotate the torso to the right in stages: lower back, mid back and shoulders and finally your head turns to look to the right. Repeat on the other side.

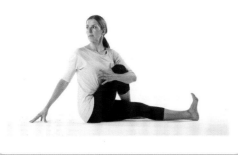

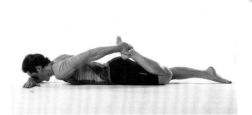

10. LYING QUAD STRETCH

Lower down onto your front. Bend your left leg and reach around for your foot. Press your hips into the floor to avoid arching your back and draw the leg closer to your buttocks. Note: if you cannot reach the foot, loop a strap or tie around it.

GOING DEEPER: LOW LUNGE WITH QUAD STRETCH

If you are comfortable bearing weight on your back knee, try performing a low lunge combined with a quad stretch. Please note: you will require flexibility to sink your hips low enough so that most of the weight on your back knee is just above the joint, on your thigh, rather than squarely on your kneecap. Do pad the back knee with a cushion or block. Perform the low lunge with your left foot in front. Now lean a little to the left, drop your left hand to the floor and bend your right leg. Reach around to hold your right foot. Shift your weight back to the centre and lift your upper body. Either hold still or do the following steps:

- Press the front of your foot into your hand.
- Draw your heel closer to your body.

If you feel balanced, end by reaching around to your foot with your right hand too, drawing back your shoulders and lifting your chest. Repeat on the other side.

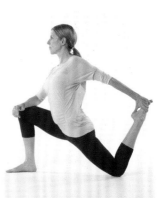

Swimming

Watch the poolside stretches of champion swimmers and their superior flexibility, particularly in the upper body, is clear. By increasing the range of movement in the shoulders, spine and ankle joints, swimmers are able to glide smoothly and create less water turbulence. Amateur swimmers can also reap performance gains through regular stretching and reduce post-swimming aches around the back and shoulders. The stretching routine below is designed with the front crawl stroke in mind, but would suit swimmers favouring other styles too.

6 Warm-Ups for Swimmers

Repeat each stretch x 4

1. DYNAMIC HEAD TURNS

Rotate your head to the right, back to the centre and over to the left. Continue to turn your head from side to side. Move in slow motion.

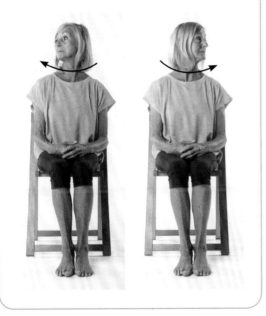

2. SWIMMING ARMS 1

Drop your fingertips onto your shoulders and 'swim' your arms by making alternate circles with your elbows. Roll your shoulders first forwards, then in a backwards motion.

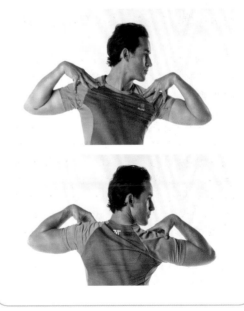

3. SWIMMING ARMS 2

'Swim' your arms mimicking a front crawl movement. Allow your upper body to rotate as you reach forwards with alternate arms. Reverse the exercise by copying the backstroke movement.

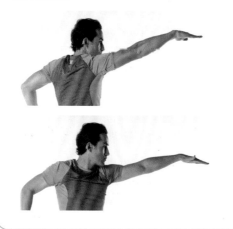

4. MID-BACK WARM-UP

Move your arms into a 90-degree position. Keep your hips and legs still and twist your upper body slowly and gently from side to side.

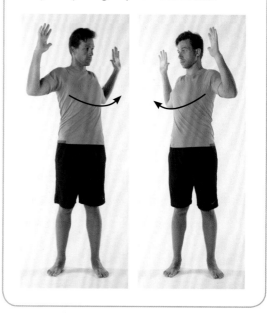

5. LEG SWING

Stand on your left leg and slowly swing your right leg back and forth. Let your arms swing freely in opposition to mimic walking or running. Repeat on the other side.

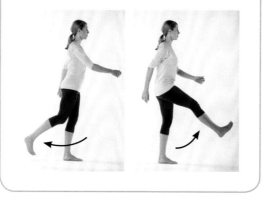

6. ANKLE ROLL

Place your hands on your hips. Stand on your left leg and lift your right foot off the floor. Rotate your foot slowly. Repeat on the other side.

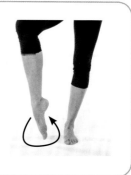

10 Post-Swim Stretches

Hold stretches for 20-30 seconds

1. FULL BODY STRETCH

Stand with your feet hip-width apart. Sweep your arms up overhead and interlink your fingers. Press your palms towards the ceiling.

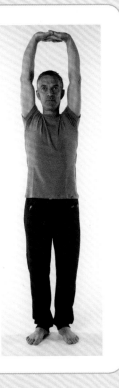

2. ASSISTED NECK EXTENSOR STRETCH

Interlink your hands behind your head. Drop your head down bringing your chin towards your chest. Do not push your head further, but let your elbows drop forwards so the weight of your arms increases the stretch.

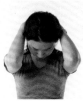

3. ASSISTED TRAPEZIUS STRETCH

Drop your head and tip it slightly to the right. Now raise your right arm up, place your right hand onto the top of your head. Gently draw your head a little deeper into the stretch. Repeat on the other side.

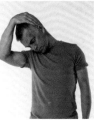

4. TRICEPS STRETCH

Stand with your feet hip-width apart. Reach up with your right arm and bend it so your hand drops behind your upper back. Use your left hand to gently draw the right elbow back. Repeat on the other side.

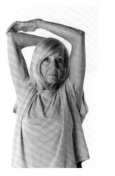

5. SHOULDER BLADE REACH STRETCH

Stand with your feet hip-width apart. Take your left arm behind your back and slide your hand up your spine towards the middle of your shoulder blades. Repeat on the other side.

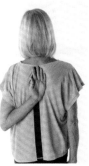

6. CHEST AND SHOULDER STRETCH

Take your arms behind your back and interlink your hands. Lift your chest, draw your shoulders back and raise your hands. Do not lean forward. Lift your hands higher to go deeper.

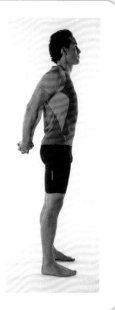

7. KNEELING BACK STRETCH WITH HOOKED THUMBS

Lower yourself down to all fours and sit on your heels. Reach your arms out in front of you. Spread your fingers and press down. Hook your thumbs together. Draw your hips away in the opposite direction, tuck your chin in and lift your mid back to go deeper.

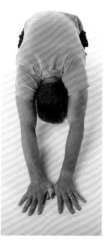

8. KNEELING SIDE STRETCH

Release your thumb hook. Walk your hands over to the right. Press your palms into the floor. Hold for 30 seconds. Walk your hands over to the left and press your palms into the floor. Hold for 30 seconds.

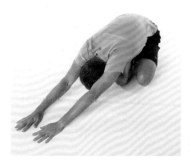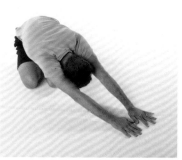

9. KNEELING TOWEL STRETCH

To gain a deeper stretch for the front of the foot and ankle, perform the kneeling position, but with a small folded towel underneath your toes.

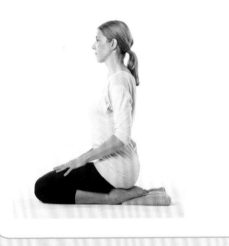

10. BASIC SEATED TWIST

Stretch your legs out in front. Bend your right leg and step it over your left. Wrap your left arm around your leg and draw your leg into your body. Drop your right fingertips behind your back and begin to rotate the torso to the right in stages: lower back, mid back and shoulders and finally your head turns to look to the right. Repeat on the other side.

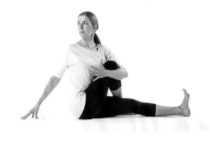

GOING DEEPER: ADVANCED TRICEPS STRETCH

This stretch combines Triceps Stretch and Shoulder Blade Reach Stretch. It is a fantastic stretch for swimmers, but does require a good degree of shoulder joint range of motion. Have a strap, tie or belt handy (hanging over the right shoulder) to aid the stretch and – as always – move in and out of the stretch slowly and with caution.

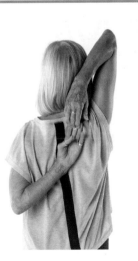

Repeat the Triceps Stretch with the right arm, but this time take your left arm behind your back and slide it up your spine. See if you can clasp your hands comfortably. If not, use the strap to bridge the gap between your hands. Don't be surprised if you can clasp on one side but not on the other; most people have a more flexible side.

Tennis and Other Racquet Sports

Flexibility is paramount for tennis, squash and badminton. A tennis player will move her joints through extreme ranges of motion. Picture the demands made of the shoulder in the serve, or the hip joint as a player steps into a deep side lunge. The lower body can also take a pounding in all racquet sports, especially the feet, calves and knees. Stretching can help players' bodies absorb the force and impact of the game, prepare their muscles for that unexpected twist or lunge to reach a shot and overcome the imbalances created by one-sided sports.

6 Warm-Ups for Racquet Sports

Repeat each stretch x 4

1. WRIST AND HAND WARMER

Interlace your fingers, palms down at chest-height. Pull your hands slightly apart as if your fingers were stuck together until you can feel some traction. Then, alternately flex and extend (bend and draw back) your wrists.

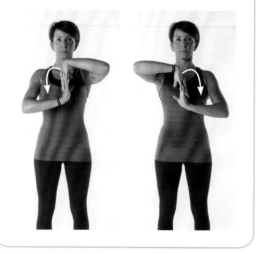

2. SWIMMING ARMS 2

'Swim' your arms mimicking a front crawl movement. Allow your upper body to rotate as you reach forwards with alternate arms. Reverse the exercise by copying the backstroke movement.

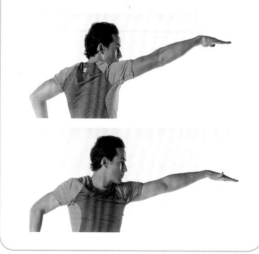

3. HEEL AND TOE ROCKING

Rock your weight back into the heels and lift your toes off the floor. Rock your weight forwards onto the balls of your feet and lift your heels off the floor.

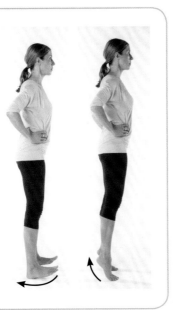

4. HEEL TAPS

Stand on your right leg. Lift your left leg up, bend it and turn your knee out. Touch your left heel with your right hand. Switch from leg to leg.

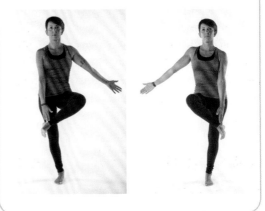

5. LUNGE WITH TWIST

Prepare to lunge but this time fold your arms and hold on to your elbows. Position the arms at chest height. As you step forwards with the right foot, rotate only your upper body to the right. Rotate your upper body to face forwards and rise back up to standing. Repeat on the other side.

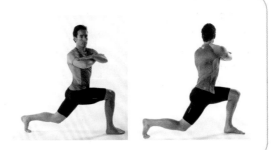

6. SPEED SKATER

Step your feet wider with your toes slightly turned outwards. Lower into a side lunge by bending your right leg and straightening your left. Sweep your left arm across your chest and drop your left elbow down. Let your upper body twist a little. Switch from side to side.

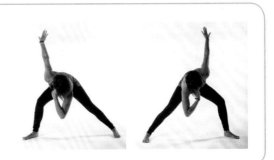

10 Post-Racquet Sports Stretches

Hold each stretch for 20–30 seconds

1. FOREARM EXTENSOR STRETCH

Stand with your right arm straight and at shoulder height. Use your left hand to gently push your right hand down. Repeat on the other side.

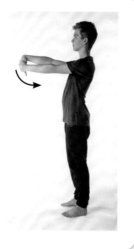

2. FOREARM FLEXOR STRETCH

Stand with your right arm straight and at shoulder height. Use your left hand to gently pull your fingers back. Repeat on the other side.

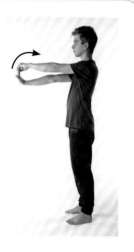

3. POSTERIOR SHOULDER STRETCH

Stand with your right arm straight and at chest height. Place your left hand behind your right elbow and draw your arm across your body. Do not rotate the torso. Repeat on the other side.

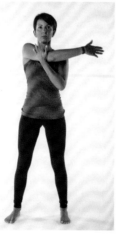

4. TRICEPS STRETCH

Stand with your feet hip-width apart. Reach up with your right arm and bend it so your hand drops behind your upper back. Use your left hand to gently draw your right elbow back.

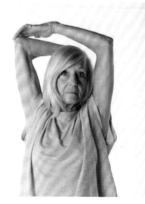

5. WIDE-LEGGED FORWARD BEND

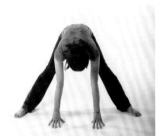

Step the feet wide and turn your toes slightly inwards. Place your hands on your hips and tip your upper body forwards, stopping when your back begins to round. Remain here, or place the hands on the floor. Let your head drop down and relax.

6. LOW LUNGE WITH TWIST

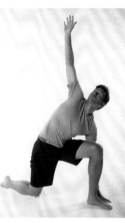

Lower yourself down to all fours. Step your left foot up in between your hands. Keep your left hand or fingertips on the floor and sweep your right arm up. Switch legs and sweep your left arm up.

7. BUTTERFLY

Sit either on the floor, or the edge of a cushion or foam block if you find it hard to straighten your spine in this position. Bring the soles of your feet together. Clasp your hands either around your feet or around your ankles and sit tall. To go deeper, keep your back straight and lean your upper body forwards.

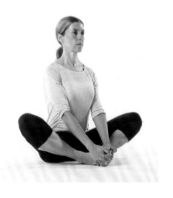

8. BASIC SEATED TWIST

Stretch your legs out in front. Bend your right leg and step it over your left. Wrap your left arm around your leg and draw your leg into your body. Drop your right fingertips behind your back and begin to rotate your torso to the right in stages: lower back, mid back and shoulders and finally your head turns to look to the right. Repeat on the other side.

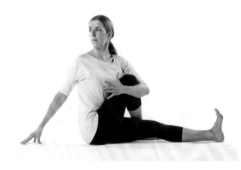

9. LYING CALF STRAP STRETCH

Lie on your back and loop a strap, belt or tie around the sole of your right foot and push your heel up. Bend your left leg and place your foot on the floor, especially if your hamstrings are tight. Stay still or move your heel from side to side. Repeat on the other side.

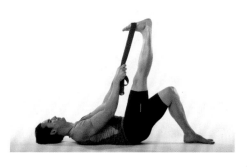

10. LYING ANKLE STRAP STRETCH

Turn the sole of your foot to face the left. Move your leg 10-20 degrees across your body. Repeat on the other side.

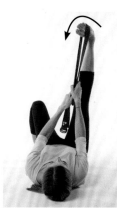

GOING DEEPER: WIDE-LEGGED TWISTS

Combine the upper body twisting action required in racquet sports with a hamstring and inner thigh stretch (Wide Legged Forward Bend). You should be able to comfortably rest your fingertips or palms on the floor in order to proceed. This technique can be done either as a static stretch, holding for 30 seconds on each side or as a dynamic flow. For the moving version, breathe in as you sweep your right arm up and breathe out as you lower it down. Repeat on the left side and move slowly from side to side.

Take your feet wide with your toes slightly turned in and rest your fingertips or palms on the floor. As you inhale, sweep your right arm up. Lower your arm down and repeat, turning to the left.

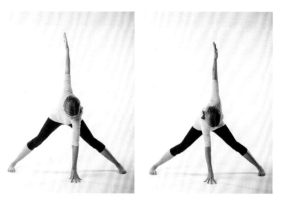

Triathlon

Due to the volume of training triathletes undertake, it is crucial to stretch regularly both to avoid niggles and injuries, but also to reap the performance benefits of owning a strong, but supple body able to withstand the rigours of all three sports. This sequence focuses on the muscles used for running, cycling and swimming, but hones in on particular triathlon injury hot spots such as the outer hip/thigh, hamstrings and calves. Additional stretches will help triathletes find comfort and form in the extreme flexed cycling position and improve shoulder range of movement for swimming.

6 Warm-Ups for Triathletes

Repeat each stretch x 4

1. HEEL AND TOE ROCKING

Rock your weight back into your heels and lift your toes off the floor. Rock your weight forwards onto the balls of your feet and lift your heels off the floor.

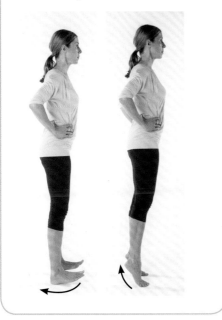

2. LEG SWING

Stand on your left leg and slowly swing your right leg back and forth. Let your arms swing freely in opposition to mimic walking or running. Switch legs.

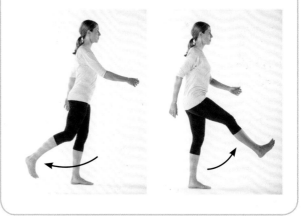

3. BACK KICKS

Stand on your left leg. Bend your right leg as if lifting your heel to your buttocks. Switch from leg to leg.

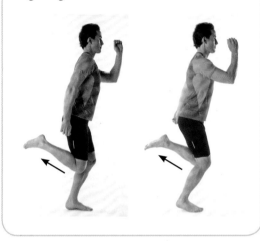

4. HEEL TAP

Stand on your right leg. Lift your left leg up, bend it and turn your knee out. Tap your left heel with your right hand. Switch from leg to leg.

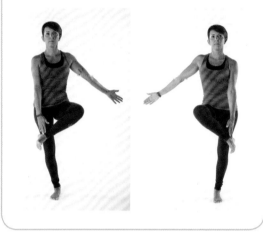

5. SWIMMING ARMS 2

'Swim' your arms mimicking a front crawl movement. Allow your upper body to rotate as you reach forwards with alternate arms. Reverse the exercise by copying the backstroke movement.

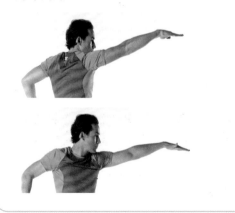

6. STANDING TWIST

Bend your knees a little and relax your arms by your sides. Twist your upper body to the right and let the arms swing around. Return to the centre and twist to the left.

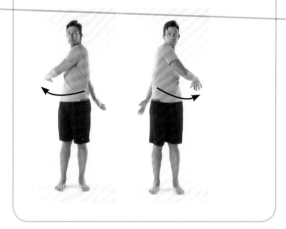

10 Post-Triathlon Stretches

Hold each stretch for 20–30 seconds

1. FULL BODY STRETCH

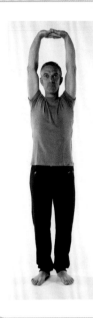

Stand with your feet hip-width apart. Sweep your arms up overhead and interlink your fingers. Press your palms towards the ceiling.

2. ASSISTED NECK EXTENSOR STRETCH

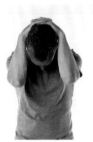

Interlink your hands behind your head. Drop your head down bringing your chin towards your chest. Do not push your head further, but let your elbows drop forwards so that the weight of your arms increases the stretch.

3. CHEST AND SHOULDER STRETCH

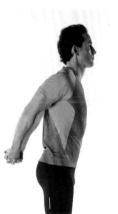

Take your arms behind your back and interlink your hands. Lift your chest, draw your shoulders back and raise your hands. Do not lean forward. Lift your hands higher to go deeper.

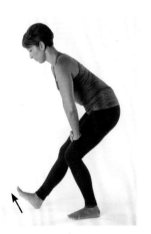

4. STANDING TOES UP STRETCH

Take a step back with your left leg. Bend your left leg and tip your upper body forwards. Lift your right toes up to roll your foot on the heel. Repeat on the other side.

5. FIGURE FOUR CHAIR

Sit on a chair with a straight back and both feet on the floor. Lift your left foot off the floor and turn your knee out. Rest your left ankle on top of your right thigh. Keeping your back straight, lean your upper body forwards a little. Lean further to up the intensity of the stretch. Repeat on the other side.

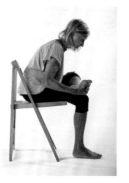

6. BASIC SEATED TWIST

Stretch your legs out in front. Bend your right leg and step it over your left. Wrap your left arm around your leg and draw your leg into your body. Drop your right fingertips behind your back and begin to rotate the torso to the right in stages: lower back, mid back and shoulders and finally your head turns to look to the right. Repeat on the other side.

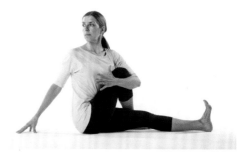

7. LOW LUNGE WITH SIDE BEND

Lower yourself down to all fours. Step your right foot up in between your hands and raise your upper body. Tuck your pelvis under. Slowly sink forwards and down into the lunge. Reach high with your left arm and lean your upper body over to the right. Repeat on the other side.

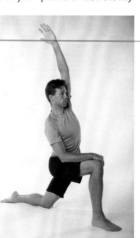

8. LIZARD

From the Lunge position, position your foot on the outside of your left hand. Sink your hips deeper into the lunge. Bend your arms or lower onto your forearms. Uncurl your back toes so the front of your foot rests on the floor. Repeat on the other side.

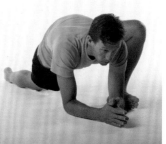

9. PIGEON

Move onto all fours. Slide your right knee up behind your right wrist. Wiggle your right foot a little over to the left. Straighten your back leg. Lower yourself slowly onto your forearms. To move deeper, lower your upper body further by resting your forehead on your stacked hands or the floor.

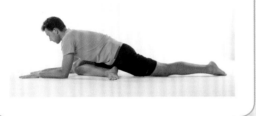

10. KNEELING BACK STRETCH WITH HOOKED THUMBS

Lower yourself down to all fours and sit on your heels. Reach your arms out in front of you. Spread your fingers and press down. Hook your thumbs together. Draw your hips away in the opposite direction, tuck your chin in and lift your mid back to go deeper.

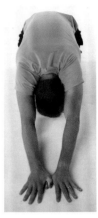

GOING DEEPER: PIGEON WITH QUAD STRETCH

Triathletes are used to multi-tasking so here's an advanced technique that ticks many boxes. Pigeon with Quad stretch will unlock tight glutes and hip flexors while providing a deep stretch for the quads. Please note: lifting the back foot places pressure on the knee joint so avoid this stretch if you have a knee injury. Ideally, you should be able to sink the hips low enough in the lunge so that when you draw the back leg in, the pressure is just above the knee joint, rather than squarely on the kneecap.

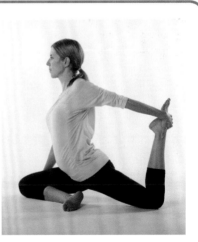

Perform Pigeon again with the right leg bent in front. Instead of lowering your upper body down to the floor, stay upright. Lean a little to the right. Bend your left leg and reach the left arm back to hold your back foot. Shift the weight back to the centre and lengthen the spine and gently draw your left leg towards you. Repeat on the other side.

Watersports

The two stretching sequences below are designed to prepare the body for the rigours of kite surfing, wakeboarding, waterskiing and windsurfing. These watersports demand good strength in the core, hands, forearms, chest, back and shoulders. Regular stretching will help enthusiasts gain flexibility so that their bodies are supple and primed for the unexpected move or fall. The aim is also to sidestep overuse injuries particularly around the elbows, lower back and knees.

6 Warm-Ups for Watersports

Repeat each stretch x 4

1. MID-BACK WARM-UP

Move your arms into a 90-degree position. Keep your hips and legs still and twist your upper body slowly and gently from side to side.

2. SWIMMING ARMS 1

Drop your fingertips onto your shoulders and 'swim' your arms by making alternate circles with your elbows. Roll your shoulders first forwards, then in a backwards motion.

3. SWIMMING ARMS 2

'Swim' your arms mimicking a front crawl movement. Allow your upper body to rotate as you reach forwards with alternate arms. Reverse the exercise by copying the backstroke movement.

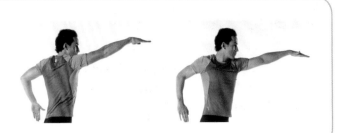

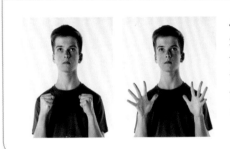

4. SQUEEZE AND SPREAD

Squeeze your hands into fists tucking the thumb in and hold for five seconds. Now spread your hands wide and hold for five seconds. *Repeat x 4.*

5. SIDE LEG SWING

Stand on your left leg and slowly swing your right leg across your body back and forth. Rest your right hand on a wall for support if required. Switch legs.

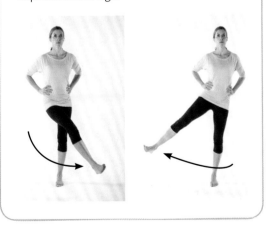

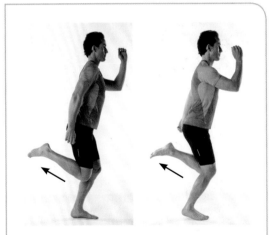

6. BACK KICKS

Stand on your left leg. Bend your right leg as if lifting your heel to your buttocks. Switch from leg to leg.

10 Post-Watersport Stretches

Hold each stretch for 20–30 seconds

1. FINGER STRETCHING

Spread your fingers wide. Gently draw back each finger one by one holding for a few seconds.

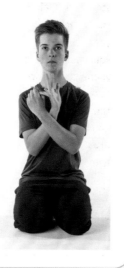

2. FOREARM EXTENSOR STRETCH

Stand with your right arm straight and at shoulder height. Gently push your right hand down. Repeat on the other side.

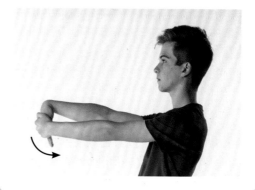

3. FOREARM FLEXOR STRETCH

Stand with your right arm straight and at shoulder height. Use your left hand to gently pull the fingers back. Repeat on the other side.

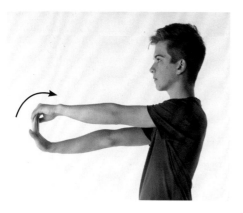

4. POSTERIOR SHOULDER STRETCH

Stand with your right arm straight and at chest height. Place your left hand behind your right elbow and draw your arm across your body. Do not rotate the torso. Repeat on the other side.

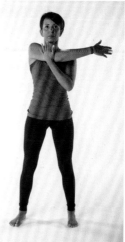

5. TRICEPS STRETCH

Stand with your feet hip-width apart. Reach up with your right arm and bend it so your hand drops behind your upper back. Use your left hand to gently draw your right elbow back. Repeat on the other side.

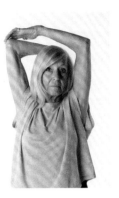

6. ASSISTED NECK EXTENSOR STRETCH

Stand tall. Interlink your hands behind your head. Drop your head, tuck your chin in and let your elbows drop forwards so the weight of the arms increases the stretch. Now begin to let your spine round until you feel the stretch spread down to your upper back. Uncurl slowly to standing and release your arms.

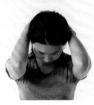

7. LOW LUNGE WITH SIDE BEND

Lower yourself down to all fours. Step your right foot up in between your hands and raise your upper body. Tuck your pelvis under. Slowly sink forwards and down into the lunge. Reach high with your left arm and lean your upper body over to the right. Repeat on the other side.

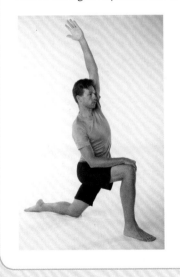

8. FIGURE FOUR SITTING

Sit on the floor or on a mat with your legs bent. Lift your right foot off the floor and turn your knee out. Rest your right ankle on top of your left thigh. Stay here or lift both feet off the floor and draw both legs in towards you. Hold behind your front thigh or clasp your front shin. Repeat on the other side.

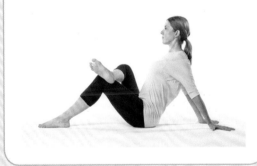

9. HAMSTRING STRAP STRETCH

Lie on your back and loop a strap, belt or tie around the sole of the right foot. Bend your left leg and place your foot on the floor, especially if your hamstrings are tight. Straighten your right leg or bend it a little. Repeat on the other side.

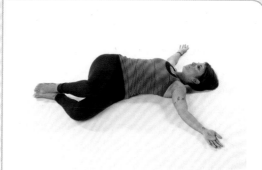

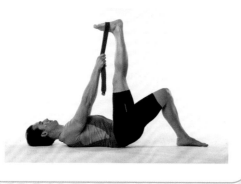

10. BASIC LYING TWIST

Drop your feet to the floor. Stretch your arms out shoulder-height, palms facing upwards. Lower both legs down to the floor on the left side and relax them.

GOING DEEPER: THE RACK STRETCH

This stretch targets the 'gripping' muscles such as the shoulders, chest and forearms used to waterski, windsurf or kitesurf. It is easily adjusted so can be made as deep or gentle as required, but avoid The Rack if you have a shoulder injury.

Move to a seated position and straighten your legs. Take your hands behind your back, fingers pointing away, and press them into the floor. Lift your chest, but keep your chin tucked in. Squeeze your shoulder blades together. To go deeper, repeat, but with your hands either close together and/or further away.

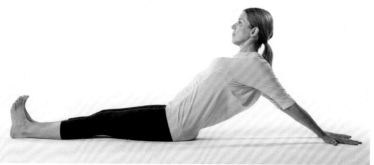

Weight Training

Observe a weightlifter drop into a deep squat and its clear to see how important it is to be both supple and strong, not just in the calves, inner thighs and hamstrings, but the lower back and shoulders, in order to achieve a strong and safe lifting position. Intense lifting with heavy weights can quickly reduce range of motion, but regular flexibility training will counter this and also benefit those working with smaller free weights and kettlebells by ensuring that they stay supple and resistant to injury.

6 Warm-Ups for Weight Training

Repeat each stretch x 4

1. KNEE CIRCLE
Stand with your feet together. Bend your legs and place your hands on your knees. Make circles with your knees.

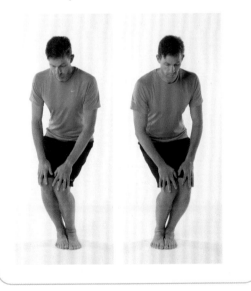

2. HIP CIRCLE
Place your hands on your hips and make large, smooth circles with your hips keeping a slight bend in your knees.

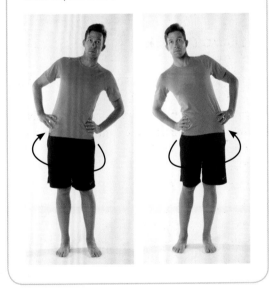

3. LEG SWING

Stand on your left leg and slowly swing your right leg back and forth. Let your arms swing freely in opposition to mimic walking or running. Switch legs.

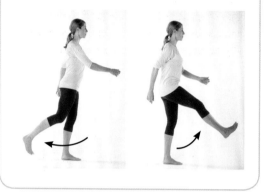

4. LUNGES

Place your hands on your hips. Take a large step forwards with your right leg and bend your knee to a 90-degree angle, ensuring your ankle is either directly over, or just behind your knee. Simultaneously drop your back knee down so that it hovers above the floor. Step back to standing. Switch from leg to leg.

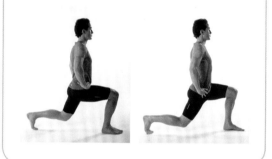

5. SUMO SQUATS

Place your hands by your sides. Step your feet wide with your toes slightly turned outwards. Bend both legs and lower into a squat checking that your knees are aligned with your second toes and your toes are just visible in the squat. Rise back up to a standing position.

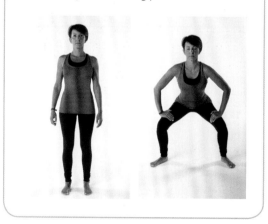

6. SWIMMING ARMS 1

Drop your fingertips onto your shoulders and 'swim' your arms by making alternate circles with your elbows. Roll your shoulders first forwards, then in a backwards motion.

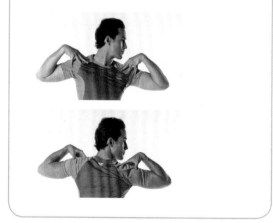

10 Post-Weight Training Stretches

Hold each stretch for 20–30 seconds

1. TRICEPS STRETCH

Stand with your feet hip-width apart. Reach up with your right arm and bend it so your hand drops behind your upper back. Use your left hand to gently draw your right elbow back. Repeat on the other side.

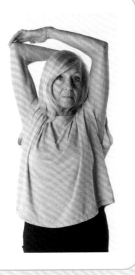

2. OVERHEAD STRAP STRETCH

Stand with your feet hip-width apart. Raise your strap, tie or belt overhead with your hands wide. Bend your arms until they form a 90-degree angle and draw your elbows back.

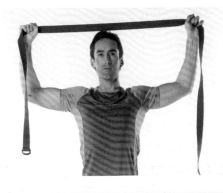

3. CHEST AND SHOULDER STRETCH

Take your arms behind your back. Interlink your hands or hold onto a strap. Lift your chest, draw your shoulders back and raise your hands. Do not lean forward. Lift your hands higher to go deeper.

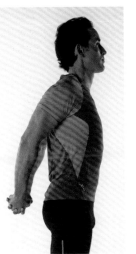

4. WIDE-LEGGED FORWARD BEND

Step your feet wide and turn your toes slightly inwards. Place your hands on your hips and tip your upper body forwards, stopping when your back begins to round. Remain here, or place your hands on the floor. Let your head drop down and relax.

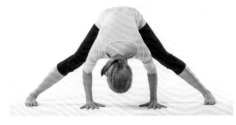

5. LOW LUNGE WITH SIDE BEND

Lower yourself down to all fours. Step your right foot up in between your hands and raise your upper body. Push your hips forwards. Slowly sink forwards and down into the lunge. Reach high with your left arm and lean your upper body over to the right. Repeat on the other side.

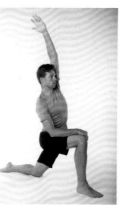

6. ACHILLES SQUAT STRETCH

Stand with your feet hip-width apart and toes facing forwards. Bend your legs and lower down into a squatting position. Rest your fingertips on the floor in front for balance if necessary.

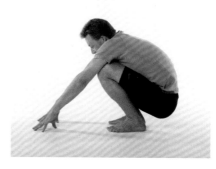

7. KNEELING BACK STRETCH WITH HOOKED THUMBS

Lower yourself down to all fours and sit on your heels. Reach your arms out in front of you. Spread your fingers and press down. Hook your thumbs together. Draw your hips away in the opposite direction, tuck your chin in and lift your mid back to go deeper.

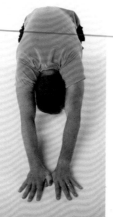

8. KNEELING SIDE STRETCH

Release your thumb hook. Walk your hands over to the right. Press your palms into the floor. Hold for 30 seconds. Walk your hands over to the left and press your palms into the floor. Hold for 30 seconds.

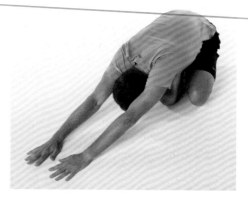

9. ROUNDED BACK STRETCH

Sit with your legs bent and feet on the floor. Clasp your hands around the back of your thighs. Round your back, let your head drop down and lean back.

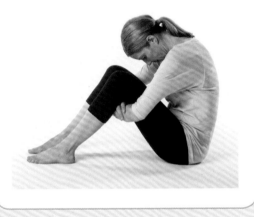

10. SEATED TWIST

Stretch your legs out in front. Bend your left leg and step it over your right. Wrap your right arm around your leg and draw it into your body. Drop your left fingertips behind your back and begin to rotate your torso to the left in stages: lower back, mid back and shoulders and finally your head turns to look to the left. Repeat on the other side.

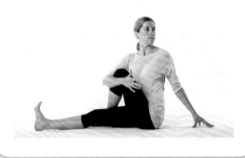

GOING DEEPER: WIDE-LEGGED BACK STRETCH

This stretch will lengthen the lifting muscles in your back while simultaneously stretching the hamstrings and inner thighs. Ensure that you can comfortably perform a Wide Legged Forward Bend (page 85) with your hands resting on the floor under each shoulder. The trick to this technique is to have very little weight resting on your hands so lean back a little to shift your weight onto your heels.

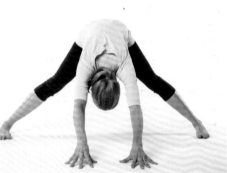

From the Wide-Legged Forward Bend position, start to move your fingertips forwards until your arms straighten. Continue to lean back onto the heels a little until you feel a stretch in your back. To deepen this back stretch, tuck your chin in and round your back slightly.

Acknowledgements

Such a visual book demanded outstanding models and I'm so grateful for Rory Spicer, Jianhua Liang, Ian Shaw, Lilly Morgado, Rosie Master and my husband Tom Williamson for providing their time, energy and a willingness to be bent into a variety of shapes for the camera. My three children; Lauren Skye, Finlay and Cameron, along with the lovely Eliza Granville, stepped in to shoot the Stretches for Children and Stretches for Teenagers sequences as well as the Wrists and Hands chapter, and all deserve a special mention. Thank you also to Sarah Connelly, my editor at Bloomsbury, for being calm, professional and logging and labelling the images so efficiently. A final dedication must go to the laid-back Grant Pritchard who shot 750-something perfect photos without raising an eyebrow. It was fun working with you and I hope you picked up a stretch or two for your lower back.

Index